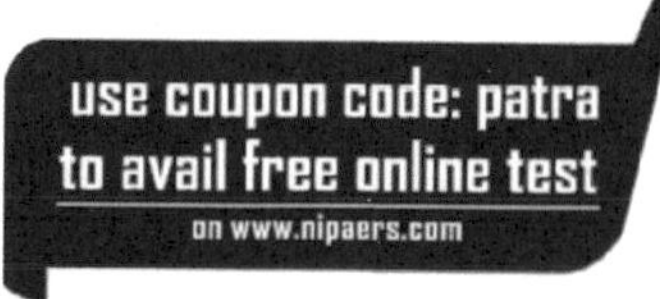

MCQs ON VETERINARY MEDICINE

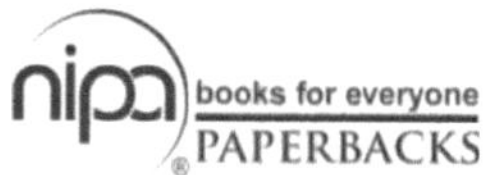

NIPA GENX ELECTRONIC RESOURCES & SOLUTIONS P. LTD.
New Delhi-110 034

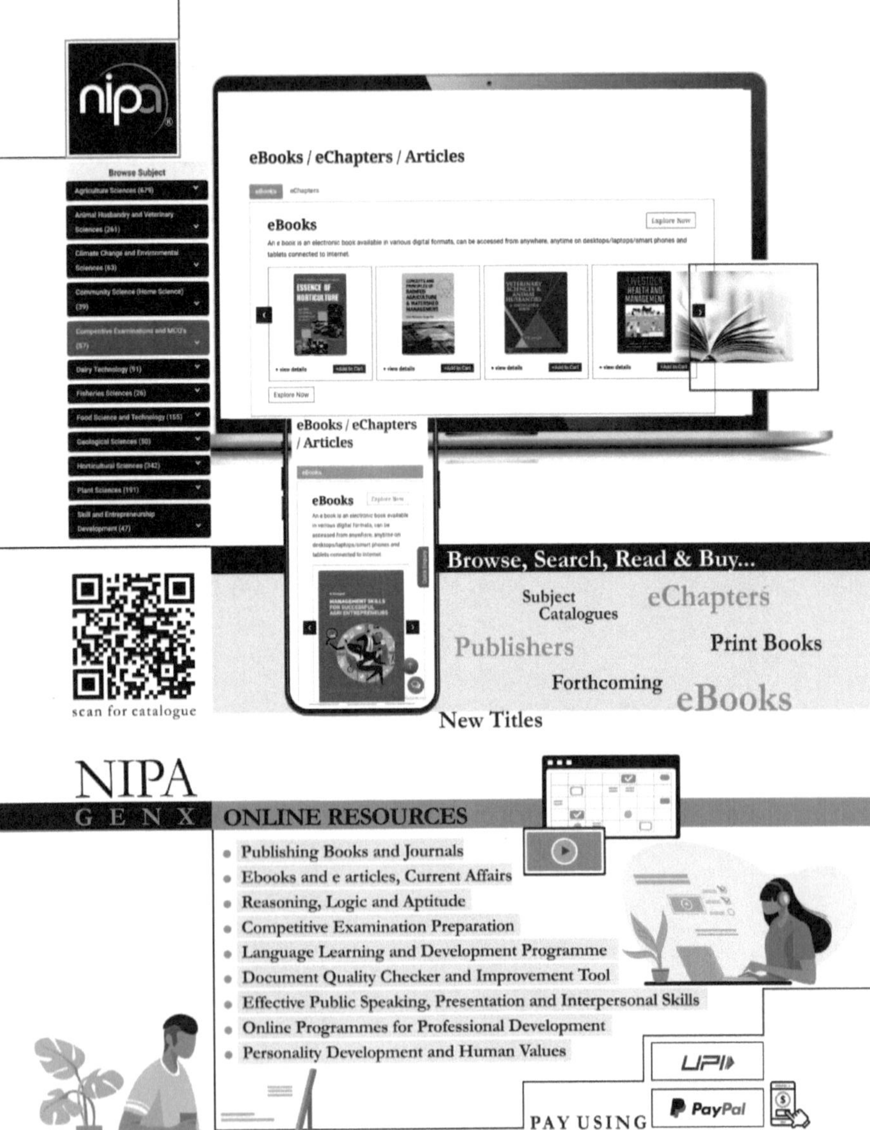

nipa
Browse Subject
Agriculture Sciences (679)
Animal Husbandry and Veterinary Sciences (261)
Climate Change and Environmental Sciences (63)
Community Science (Home Science) (39)
Dairy Technology (91)
Fisheries Sciences (26)
Food Science and Technology (155)
Geological Sciences (30)
Horticultural Sciences (342)
Plant Sciences (191)
Skill and Entrepreneurship Development (47)
eBooks / eChapters / Articles
eBooks
An e book is an electronic book available in various digital formats, can be accessed from anywhere, anytime on desktops/laptops/smart phones and tablets connected to internet.
Explore Now
scan for catalogue
Browse, Search, Read & Buy...
Subject Catalogues
eChapters
Publishers
Print Books
Forthcoming
eBooks
New Titles
NIPA
GENX
ONLINE RESOURCES
Publishing Books and Journals
Ebooks and e articles, Current Affairs
Reasoning, Logic and Aptitude
Competitive Examination Preparation
Language Learning and Development Programme
Document Quality Checker and Improvement Tool
Effective Public Speaking, Presentation and Interpersonal Skills
Online Programmes for Professional Development
Personality Development and Human Values
PAY USING
UPI
PayPal

MCQs ON VETERINARY MEDICINE

Ramesh Chandra Patra, PhD
NAVS Fellow (2016), IAAVR Fellow (2016), ISVM Fellow (2007)
BOYSCAST Fellow (USA), DBT CREST Fellow (UK)
DBT Overseas Associate and Endeavour Research Fellow (Australia)
Professor and Head, Department of Veterinary Clinical Medicine
Former Dean, College of Veterinary Science & Animal Husbandry and
Dean of Research, Odisha University of Agriculture & Technology (OUAT)
Bhubaneswar, Odisha, India

Debiprasanna Das, PhD
Diplomate, Indian College of Veterinary Pathology
Assistant Professor, Department of Veterinary Pathology
College of Veterinary Science & Animal Husbandry,
Odisha University of Agriculture & Technology (OUAT)
Bhubaneswar, Odisha, India

Rajasri Sahoo, PhD
UGC BSR Fellow
Lecturer, Banki Autonomus College
Cuttack, Odisha, India

Biswa Ranjan Jena
University Gold Medalist (OUAT), ICAR-SRF
"Shri Lal Bahadur Shastri VIPM best" PG Thesis Awardee
Bhubaneswar, Odisha, India

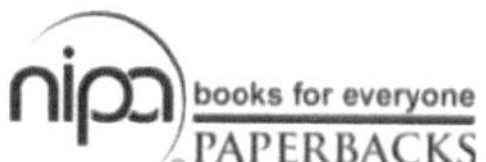

NIPA GENX ELECTRONIC RESOURCES & SOLUTIONS P. LTD.
New Delhi-110 034

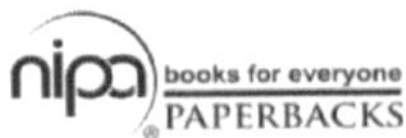

NIPA GENX ELECTRONIC RESOURCES & SOLUTIONS P. LTD.

101,103, Vikas Surya Plaza, CU Block
L.S.C.Market, Pitam Pura, New Delhi-110 034
Ph : +91 11 27341616, 27341717, 27341718
E-mail:newindiapublishingagency@gmail.com
www: www.nipabooks.com

For customer assistance, please contact
Phone: + 91-11-27 34 17 17 Fax: + 91-11- 27 34 16 16
E-Mail: feedbacks@nipabooks.com

ISBN: 978-93-94490-23-9

Composed and Designed by NIPA.

Preface

We envisage to to publish a book containing multiple choice questions and answer on the subject "Veterinary Medicine" to facilitate students appearing competitive examination to assess their knowledge level after studying the chapters in Veterinary Medicine. This book contains chapter-wise questions and answers, followed by question sets from whole course of Veterinary Medicine.

The first author of this book Dr R C Patra had initial acquaintance to animal husbandry practices in a rural set up during his school days from where he developed interest in veterinary profession. His admission to Undergraduate course in Veterinary Science and Animal Husbandry in the year 1984 cherished his school days interest. Subsequently, he pursued his master and doctoral degree in the discipline of Veterinary Medicine in the premier national institute, ICAR-Indian Veterinary Research Institute. He started his professional career as a grass root level field veterinarian for animal healthcare services for Odisha state. His academic career started with joining Indian Council of Agricultural Research as Agricultural Research Scientist. During this period, he availed BOYSCAST fellowship to pursue post-doctoral research in John Hopkins University, USA. He moved to his Alma-matter as Professor of Veterinary Medicine after serving for almost one and half decade in ICAR.

Introduction of Minimum Standard of Veterinary Education (MSVE) by Veterinary Council of India (VCI) ignited the first author to write a reader friendly concise book on Veterinary Clinical Medicine by referring standard books, research articles and utilizing his writing and teaching skill, and knowledge gained from clinical practice for more than two decades. The publication of the book prompted us to write a book consisting of multiple choice questions and answers on Veterinary Medicine. Along with Co-authors Dr D.P. Das, Dr Rajasri Sahoo and Dr Biswa Ranjan Jena,and chapter-wise expert contributors, multiple choice questions were synthesized for the benefit of the students appearing competitive examinations. As a senior author, I extend my gratitude to my beloved teachers and express profuse thanks to my loving students, colleagues and friends, and the publisher whose constant inspiration and support helped to complete this publication. This book will be very much helpful to the students preparing for Senior Research Fellowship, National Eligibility Test and Junior Research Fellowship, and other competitive examinations.

Contents

List of Contributors

Expert	Title of the Chapter
Dr G. R. Jena Assistant Professor in Veterinary Medicine	Diseases of Urinary System
Dr Basanti Jena Assistant Professor in Animal Reproduction Gynaecology and Obstetrics	Diseases of Neonates
Dr S. K. Senapati Associate Professor in Veterinary Medicine	Emergency Medicine and Critical Care
Dr Rajasri Sahoo Lecturer in Botany	Alternative Medicine in Animal Diseases Management
Dr S. Meher Assistant Professor on Veterinary Medicine	Diseases of Blood and Blood Forming Organs
Dr Biswa Ranjan Jena Doctoral Student in Veterinary Medicine	Infectious Such as Bacterial, Viral and Parasitic Diseases and Epidemiology

1

History and Scope of Veterinary Medicine

1 Study of animal diseases at patient bed side for diagnosis, prognosis, monitoring and treatment comes under

a) Veterinary Epidemiology b) Preventive Medicine

c) Veterinary Jurisprudence d) Veterinary Clinical Medicine

2 The term "medicine" has come from Latin word MEDIR, that means

a) Heal b) Treatment

c) Diagnosis d) Examination of the patient

3 The Veterinarian has to interact with the patient owner in non-technical language to achieve the objective of

a) Proper history taking

b) Payment of user fee

c) Clinical Examination of the patient

d) Examination of the environment

4 Which of the following does not come under the role of Veterinarian

a) Creation of public awareness about zoonotic diseases

b) Epidemiological studies on animal diseases

c) Extension activities in the field of livestock health

d) Issue of legal notices in veterolegal cases involving animals

5 The institutes imparting Veterinary education and recognized by Veterinary Council of India can revise the syllabus to certain extent as per

a) Interest of the students b) National need

c) Regional needs d) International need

6 Who is considered as an expert in animal healing in Mesopotamia, during 3000 BC

a) Abraham Lincoln b) Joseph Leister

c) Urluganledinna d) A. Flemming

7 The treatment of animal diseases has been described in books written by

a) Salihotra b) Charaka

c) Palikapaya d) All of the above

8 Who among the following Pandavas had expertise in treatment and management of horses

a) Yudhisthira b) Arjuna

c) Nakula d) Sahadeva

9 Who is known as the father of Veterinary Medicine

a) Urlugiledinna b) Robert Koch

c) Hyppocrates d) Lewis Pasture

10 Viruses could be detected by electron microscope way back in the decade

a) 1840's b) 1920's

c) 1960's d) 1940's

11 The first Veterinary School was established in the year 1761 by Claude Boungelat in France in the city of

a) Paris b) Lyon

c) Cannes d) Strasbourg

12 In India, a Veterinary Training School started at Pune in

a) 1962 b) 1862

c) 1926 d) 1826

13 The first Veterinary College was established in India in the year 1884 in the city of

a) Kolkatta b) Madras

c) Patna d) Mumbai

14 Which of the following periods is considered as golden age for Veterinary Profession because of tremendous progress of Veterinary Science

a) 1845 - 1855 b) 1885 - 1925

c) 1945 - 1985 d) 1995 - 2020

15 The second viral disease that has been eradicated from India is

a) Foot and Mouth disease b) Rabies

c) Rinderpest d) Hog Cholera

16 The buffalo population in India constitute what percentage of world population as per animal census, 2011

a) 15% b) 35%

c) 37% d) 57%

17 Which of the followings is not a wasting disease?

a) Tuberculosis b) Johnes disease

c) Hookworm infestation d) Rabies

18 The role played by today's Veterinarian does not include

a) Ensuring food safety b) Border control and quarantine

c) Environmental Protection d) None of the above

19 Penicillin was invented by

a) Alexander Flemming b) Edward Jain

c) Edward Jenner d) Robert Koch

20 The viral disease eradicated from India is

a) Rinderpest b) PPR

c) Bird flu d) Swine flu

Answer Key

1	d	**2**	a	**3**	a	**4**	d	**5**	c	**6**	c	**7**	d	**8**	c	**9**	c	**10**	d
11	b	**12**	b	**13**	d	**14**	c	**15**	c	**16**	d	**17**	d	**18**	d	**19**	a	**20**	a

2

Concept of Animal Disease

1 Health is defined as a state

a) Where all body system function normally

b) Absence of disease

c) Activities continue within normal physiological limits

d) All of the above

2 The concept of health and disease can be described in the following category

a) Health as normality b) Health as homeostasis

c) Health as biological function d) All of the above

3 When there is no recognizable and visible abnormalities, no apparent signs of illness, then the disease is classified as

a) Clinical b) Sub-clinical

c) Acute d) Sub-acute

4 Which of the following diseases are considered as infectious diseases

a) Metabolic diseases b) Deficiency diseases

c) Allergy induced diseases d) Diseases caused by mites

5 When the disease process is slow, the ill effects are minimal and the prognosis is favourable, it is classified as

a) Severe b) Moderate

c) Mild d) None of the above

6 Diagnosis of a disease includes

a) Determination of specific cause

b) Abnormality of structure and function

c) Clinical manifestations associated with abnormality

d) All of the above

7 Manifestation of disease or disorder that is felt by the patient himself is called

a) Sign b) Symptoms

c) Pathognomonic sign d) Syndrome

8 A group or combination of clinical signs which are indicative of a particular disease is called

a) Pathognomonic sign b) Symptoms
c) Syndrome d) Clinical sign

9 Forecasting of disease outcome based on clinical and pathological alterations, in a disease process and response to continuing treatment is called

a) Diagnosis b) Symptoms
c) Prognosis d) Management

10 The process of confirming a particular disease, from other diseases producing almost similar clinical signs is called

a) Diagnosis b) Syndrome recognition
c) Differential diagnosis d) Prognosis

11 Making a diagnosis of the disease involves detailed clinical examination that consists of

a) Examination of Animal b) History taking
c) Examination of the environment d) All of the above

12 Anamnesis includes

a) Patient data b) Disease history
c) Management History d) All of the above

13 The clue in cases of organophosphate poisoning is better appreciated by

a) History taking b) Examination of the environment
c) Patient data d) Management history

14 Observation of clinical sign from a distance comes under

a) Examination of the environment b) History taking
c) Examination of the animal d) None of the above

15 Which component of clinical examination has major importance in animal practice for diagnosis of the disease

a) History taking b) Laboratory test
c) Examination of the environment d) Physical examination

Answer Key

1 d **2** d **3** b **4** d **5** c **6** d **7** b **8** c **9** c **10** c
11 d **12** d **13** b **14** c **15** a

3

Diagnosis and Differential Diagnosis of Animal Diseases

1 Diagnosis of a disease includes
   a) Determination of specific cause
   b) Abnormality of structure and functions produced by causative agent
   c) Clinical manifestation associated with the abnormality
   d) All of the above

2 Manifestation of a particular disorder in an animal which is observed by the clinician, attendant or owner is called as
   a) Signs   b) Symptoms
   c) Syndrome   d) Lesion

3 Specific signs observed in a particular disease that provides sufficient clues for making a diagnosis is called
   a) Symptoms   b) Pathognomic signs
   c) Pathogronomic lesions   d) Syndrome

4 Prognosis of a disease is based on
   a) Clinical observations of the animals
   b) Clinicopathological alterations in a disease process
   c) Response to continuing treatment
   d) All of the above

5 History taking or anamnesis comprises of
   a) Patient data   b) Disease history
   c) Management History   d) All of the above

6 General and physical examination of a patient includes
   a) Examination from a distance
   b) Examination using palpation, percussion and ascultation
   c) Examination of body part
   d) All of the above

7 Rumination for re-mastication of regurgitated food is observed as

a) Flank movement

b) Jaw movement

c) Swallowing of food

d) All of the above

8 Site of taking pulse in animals are

a) Middle coccygeal artery and facial artery in cattle

b) Facial artery in horse and mule

c) Femoral artery of sheep and goats

d) All of the above

9 Paralysis occuring in Rabies is

a) Ascending Anterior b) Descending Anterior

c) Ascending posterior d) Descending posterior

10 The word endoscopy is derived from

a) Latin word b) Greek word

c) German word d) None of the above

11 Device used to measure cardiac function during excercise in horses

a) Phonocardiography b) Telemetric ECG

c) Both (a) and (b) d) None of the above

12 Device used for recording cardiac sounds and murmers using chest surface microphone is

a) ECG b) Telemetric ECG

c) Phonocardiograph d) None of the above

13 Which of the following is /are example of non-invasive diagnostic techniques

a) Radiography b) Ultrasonography

c) Both (a) and (b) d) None of theabove

14 MRI uses the followings to create images

a) Radio waves b) UV rays

c) Strong magnetic field d) Both (a) and (c)

15 In which year Scintigraphy was produced in Veterinary Medicine

a) 1957 b) 1970

c) 1980 d) 2000

16 Which of these diagnostic techniques use Gamma Camera

a) Radiography b) Ultrasonography

c) Scintigraphy d) None of the above

17 Principle used in Scintigraphy is/are

a) Principle of X-ray b) Radioactivity

c) Both (a) and (b) d) None of the above

18 Methods for physical examination includes

a) Palpation b) Percussion

c) Auscultation d) All of the above

19 Palpation reveals the information on

a) Pain, oedema, consistency

b) Consistency, sound from different critical moist rates

c) Heart sound, pulse rate

d) Fluid accumulation

20 Palpation finding where tissue appears solid like muscle and moves with polyatom is called

a) Hard b) Fluctuating

c) Resilient d) Doughy

21 A loud sound produced by processing organs filled with gas under pressure is called

a) Dull sound b) Tympanic sound

c) Metallic ring sound d) Resonant sound

22 What type of sound is produced by percussion of large muscles or liver as in case of hepatitis or heart affected with pericardititis

a) Ping sound

b) Dull sound

c) Resonance

d) Empty muscle sound or Absolute damping sound

23 A modified form of percussion consisting of palpation and percussion to know the consistency and boundaries of deeply situated organs is called

a) Tactile percussion b) Palpative percussion

c) Indirect percussion d) Advanced percussion

24 The word Auscultation is derived from a latin word “auscultare”which means

a) To feel
b) To listen
c) To deserve
d) None of the above

25 Vesicular lungs sound is reduced in case where

a) Chest wall is thick
b) Air content of the lungs is reduced
c) Lungs are congested passively
d) All of the above

26 Which of the followings is /are correct regarding lungs sound

a) Inspiratory vesicular lungs sound resembles with the pronaunciation of letter “V”
b) Expiratory vesicular lungs sound resembles with the pronaunciation of letter “F”
c) Tubular/ Bronchial lungs sound resembles with the pronaunciation of letter “H”
d) None of the above

27 Which of the following is true regarding body temperature

a) Varginal temperature is 1°F higher than rectal temperatures during oestrus
b) Temperature of female animals is higher than male animals
c) Temperature is directly proprotional to body weight
d) All of the above

Answer Key

1 d **2** a **3** b **4** d **5** d **6** d **7** b **8** d **9** c **10** b
11 c **12** c **13** c **14** d **15** b **16** c **17** c **18** d **19** a **20** c
21 b **22** d **23** a **24** b **25** d **26** d **27** d

4

General Systemic States

1 The changes in functioning at the cellular level and establishment of disease process is termed

a) Pathogenesis b) Virulence

c) Prognosis d) None of the above

2 Elevation of body temperature beyond the critical temperature in absence of circulating toxin in the blood vascular system and resulting from failure of thermoregulation by the hypothalamus is termed as

a) Fever b) Hyperthermia

c) Septicemia d) Toxemia

3 Two signals integrated by the thermoregulatory centre of the hypothalamus to maintain normal temperature are

a) Signals from warmth/cold receptors of skin

b) Signals from blood-bathing regions

c) Both (a) and (b)

d) None of the above

4 Which of the following is incorrect regarding hyperthermia

a) Increased thirst due to dryness of mouth

b) Heart rate is increased due to rise in blood temperature

c) Blood pressure falls due to peripheral vasodilation

d) Formation of urine and urine output increases due to increased water intake

5 Death due to hyperthermia is may be due to

a) Depression of nervous activities and respiratory centers

b) Dehydration

c) Low blood pressure

d) All of the above

6 Death occurs when the temperature reaches

a) 104 °F to 108 °F
b) 106 °F to 110 °F
c) 106 °F to 108 °F
d) 104 °F to 110 °F

7 Necropsy findings in hyperthermic animals are

a) Peripheral vasodialation
b) Slow blood clotting
c) Rigor motis and purification sets early
d) All of the above

8 Factors enhancing susceptibility to hypothermia are

a) Low birth weight
b) Prematurely altered young ones
c) Poor body condition
d) All of the above

9 Which of the following is correct regarding the treatment of hypothermia

a) Severely hypothermic animals should not be kept in a shower/bath
b) Lactated Ringer's solution should not be given
c) Cold fluid administration should be avoided
d) All of the above

10 Pyrexia/Fever word is derived from

a) Latin word "febris"
b) Greek word "pyretos"
c) Both (a) and (b)
d) None of the above

11 Hyperthermia associated with toxemia is termed as

a) Fever
b) Septicemia
c) Heat stroke
d) Septic fever

12 Which of the following is not an endogenous pyrogen

a) TNF-α
b) IL-1
c) IL-6
d) LPS of gram -ve bacteria

13 Which of these enzymes mediates the arachidonic acid pathway for the synthesis of PGE2

a) PGE2 synthase
b) PLA2
c) Cox-2
d) All of the above

14 When fever subsides within 24 to 48 hours after the onset is called as

a) True fever
b) Transient fever
c) Intermittent fever
d) Atypical fever

15 Which of the following disease shows biphasic fever

a) Canine distemper b) Louping ill

c) Strangles d) All of the above

16 Type of fever in which temperature does not rise too high and remain below 103°F is called as

a) Acute fever b) Mild fever

c) Subacute fever d) Chronic fever

17 High rise of temperature accompanied with a strong bounding pulse as observed in acute inflammatory condition is classified as

a) Periodic fever b) Asthenic fever

c) Continuous fever d) Sthenic fever

18 Second stage of fever is called as

a) Initial stage/Stadium incrementi

b) Hot stage/Stadium fastigii

c) Stage of defervescence/Stadium decrementii

d) None of the above

19 Tetanus toxin is an example of which type of toxin

a) Exotoxin b) Endotoxin

c) Enterotoxin d) None of the above

20 Factors contributing endotoxemia condition

a) Large amount of endotoxin b) Liver failes to detoxify toxins

c) Injury to intestine/ enteritis d) All of the above

21 Toxins of which bacteria is used to induce experimental Endotoxemia

a) Clostridium species b) *E. coli*

c) Pasteurella d) Salmonella

22 Excessive accumulation of fluid in tissue spaces caused by a disturbance in the mechanism of fluid interchange between capillaries, tissue spaces and lymphatic vessels is called as

a) Hydrocele b) Edema

c) Ascitis d) Blisters

23 Normal rate of administration of fluids in calories is

a) 90 ml/kgbw/hr (I/v) b) 3.5 lit/hr (I/v)

c) 10-12 lit/hr (I/v) d) 12-15 lit/hr (I/v)

Answer Key

1	a	**2**	b	**3**	c	**4**	d	**5**	a	**6**	c	**7**	d	**8**	d	**9**	d	**10**	c
11	a	**12**	d	**13**	d	**14**	b	**15**	d	**16**	c	**17**	d	**18**	b	**19**	a	**20**	d
21	b	**22**	b	**23**	b														

5

Dehydration, Electrolyte and Acid Base Imbalance

1 What percentage of body weight is intracellular water

a) 60 b) 40

c) 20 d) 15

2 The force that maintains inter compartmental distribution of water is called

a) Hydrostatic force b) Osmotic force

c) Oncotic force d) All of the above

3 Rupture of the urinary bladder in the neonatal foals is associated with which of the following conditions

a) Hypernatremia b) Hyponatremia

c) Hypochloremia d) Both (a) and (b)

4 Chloride concentration variation is

a) Directly proportional to sodium concentration

b) Inversely proportional to bicarbonate concentration

c) Both (a) and (b)

d) None of the above

5 What is the serum concentration of potassium?

a) 6m Eq/L b) 4 m Eq/L

c) 2m Eq/L d) 5m Eq/L

6 Which of the following is mainly an intracellular electrolyte

a) Sodium b) Potassium

c) Chloride d) Bicarbonate

7 Decreased serum concentration of potassium is called as

a) Hyponatremia b) Hypokalemia

c) Hypocalcemia d) Hypopotamia

8 Administration of insulin or glucose and rapid administration of sodium bicarbonate in large dose can result into

a) Alkalosis and hypokalemia b) Alkalosis and hyperkalemia

c) Acidosis and hypokalemia d) Acidosis and hyperkalemia

9 Which of the following is/are responsible for the excretion of excess acids

a) Liver, Kidneys b) Lungs, Kidneys

c) Lungs, Liver d) None of the above

10 Which of the following is used as a marker of blood volatile acid level

a) PO2 b) PCO2

c) Both (a) and (b) d) None of the above

11 Organ responsible for the regulation of blood base is

a) Liver b) Lungs

c) Kidney d) Stomach

12 Hyperdemic shock develops when there is a deficit in blood volume of

a) ≥ 15% b) ≥ 12%

c) ≥ 10% d) ≥ 20%

13 Type of fluid therapy designed to replenish existing fluid deficits which usually requires replacement of both water and electrolytes is called

a) Maintenance fluid therapy b) Replacement fluid therapy

c) Emergency fluid therapy d) None of the above

14 Maximum fluid administration rate in dogs is

a) 60 ml/kg/hr b) 90 ml /kg/hr

c) 70 ml/kg/hr d) 100 ml/kg/hr

15 During anaesthsia, the normal fluid administration rate in dogs and cats is

a) 5-10 ml/kg/hr b) 15-20 ml

c) 10-20 ml/kg/hr d) 20-25 ml/kg/hr

16 Dry mucous membrane, considerable loss of skin turgor and eyes refracted indicate ______% dehydration

a) 4-5% b) 6-7%

c) 8-10% d) 10-12%

17 Major effectors of effective circulating volume is/are

a) Sympathetic nervous system b) Angiotension II

c) Renal sodium excretion d) All of the above

18 Which of the following is correct

a) Hypovolemia causes an increase in renin secretion

b) Angiotensin II causes increase in blood pressure

c) Angiotensin II causes decrease in renal sodium retention

d) All of the above

19 What is the percentage of dehydration when there is mild to moderate decreased skin turgor, dry oral mucous membranes, slight tachycardia and normal pulse pressure

a) <5

b) 5

c) 7

d) 10

20 What is the percentage of dehydration when there is marked loss of skin turgor, dry oral mucus membranes and significant signs of shock

a) 5

b) 7

c) 20

d) 10

21 In general, intravenous fluid administration is indicated in dogs and cats with ______ % dehydration

a) ≥ 5

b) ≥ 7

c) ≤ 5

d) ≤ 7

22 Total deficit Replacement volume

a) Estimated dehydration of bodyweight

b) Deficit volume + maintenance volume

c) % dehydration X bodyweight X 0.80+maintenance volume

d) Both (b) and (c)

23 _________ is the source of osmotic pressure in plasma

a) Antithrombin

b) Albumin

c) Platelets

d) All of the above

24 What is the fluid of choice in case of Adrenocortical insufficiency

a) Ringer's Lactate

b) 0.9% NaCl+ KCl

c) 0.9% NaCl

d) 5% Dextrose

25 Which of the followings is an isotonic solution

a) 1.3% Sodium bicarbonate

b) 5% Sodium bicarbonate

c) 1.8% Potassium chloride

d) 25% Dextrose

Answer Key

1 b	**2** d	**3** d	**4** c	**5** b	**6** b	**7** b	**8** a	**9** b	**10** b
11 c	**12** a	**13** b	**14** b	**15** c	**16** c	**17** d	**18** d	**19** c	**20** d
21 b	**22** d	**23** b	**24** c	**25** a					

6

Diseases of Digestive System

1 True vomiting is seen in

a) Pseudoruminants b) Monogastric animal

c) Ruminants d) All

2 Diarrhoea is generally associated with

a) Alkalosis b) Loss of bicarbonate ions

c) Acidosis d) Both (b) and (c)

3 Elimination of less quantity of faeces with normal consistency is called as

a) Constipation b) Parcopresis

c) Scant faeces d) Anismus

4 Blood in vomitus is called

a) Haematemesis b) Haemoptysis

c) Haematochezia d) Haemorrhoids

5 Partial loss of appetite is called as

a) Anorexia b) Inappetance

c) Bulimia nervosa d) Bingeing

6 Inflammation of oral mucosa is called as

a) Glossitis b) Stomatitis

c) Gingivitis d) Palatitis

7 Polaprezinc drug is

a) Chelated form of zinc and L-carnosine

b) Chelated form of Zinc and Ascorbic acid

c) Chelated form of Zn and L-carnosine

d) Chelated form of Zn and propionic acid

8 Polaprezinc is used for effective treatment of

a) Alkali induced stomatitis b) Plicamycin induced stomatitis

c) Oxallic acid induced stomatitis d) Acetic acid induced stomatitis

9 Bluish color teeth in young animals is due to deficiency of

a) Fluoride b) Magnesium

c) Oxallic acid induced stomatitis d) Acetic acid stomatitis

10 Foul smelling from mouth is called as

a) Ketoacidosis b) Halitosis

c) Pityriasis d) None

11 A hereditary condition, characterized by opening in the hard palate between mouth and nasal cavity and associated with difficulty in prehension and mastication of the food, is

a) Harelip condition b) Split lip condition

c) Cleft palate d) All of the above

12 Deficiency of which of the following vitamin leads to affection of the Salivary gland?

a) Vit-E b) Vit-A

c) Vit-Bcomplex d) All of the above

13 "Cud dropping" condition is associated with

a) Pharyngitis b) Pharyngeal obstruction

c) Pharyngeal paralysis d) All of the above

14 A pocket like structure and an outpouching of mucosa through the muscular layer of the oesophagus is called as

a) Guttural sac b) Oesophageal diverticulum

c) Oesophageal bag d) Oesophagial achalasia

15 Diagnosis of oesophageal diverticulum can be made by using contrast radiography with the use of

a) Iopamidol b) Ioversol

c) Barium meal d) Metrizoate

16 Failure of the smooth muscles of the oesophagus to relax, thus impeding the passage of food from mouth to stomach is called

a) Oesophagitis b) Oesophageal achalasia

c) Oesophageal diverticulum d) Oesophageal atresia

17 Haematological findings in traumatic reticulo peritonitis reveals

a) Neuropenia

b) Neutrophillia and shift to right, leucocytosis

c) Neutrophillia and shift to left, leucocytosis

d) None of the above

18 A sudden change in quantity, quality, composition of food or change in feeding time that brings about alteration in

a) Ruminal atony

b) Simple indigestion

c) Sudden change in pH of the ruminal contents due to excessive formation of ingested feed

d) All of the above

19 Hoven is also called

a) Bloat
b) Tympany
c) Peritonitis
d) Both (a) and (b)

20 Failure of eructation mechanism due to trapping of gases of fermentation as stable, persistant foam leads to

a) Pasture bloat
b) Frothy bloat
c) Primary tympany
d) All of the above

21 Failure of eructation of the free gas produced in the rumen due to esophageal obstruction is called as

a) Secondary tympany
b) Free gas bloat
c) Primary bloat
d) Both (a) and (b)

22 The cause of death regardless of any bloat condition is due to

a) Anemia
b) Oedema
c) Hypoxia
d) Dehydration

23 Acute clinical ruminal acidosis is characterized by

a) pH value less than 5 and lactic acid accumulation upto 300 mmol/L

b) Rumen microflora is dominated by Gram +ve bacteria

c) Defaunation

d) All of the above

24 Ruminal osmolarity normally ranges from

a) 120 to 150 mosm/L with roughage diet and 10-20 mosm/L with concentrate diet

b) 600 to 700 mosm/L with roughage diet and 100-200 mosm/L with concentrate diet

c) 240 to 265 mosm/L with roughage diet and 280-300 mosm/L with concentrate diet

d) None of the above

25 False milk fever is also known as

a) PPH
b) Ruminal acidosis
c) Founder
d) Both (b) and (c)

26 Common sequalae in chronic ruminal acidosis is

a) Liver abscess
b) Pneumonia
c) Ruminal parakeratosis
d) Both (a) and (b)

27 Systemic ruminal acidosis can be rectified by administration of

a) 0.2% KOH solution
b) 2.5% $NaHCO_3$ solution
c) 7.5% $NaHCO_3$ solution
d) 1% $NaHCO_3$ solution

28 For optimum ruminal fermentation, the optimum pH should be between

a) 5.5 to 6.5
b) 6.5 to 6.8
c) 6.9 to 7.3
d) 6.1 to 6.6

29 SARA (Subacute Ruminal Acidosis) most common in

a) Sheep
b) Goat
c) High yielding cows
d) Heifers

30 Severe grain induced SARA is dominated by

a) Streptococcus bovis & Megaspharaelsdenil
b) Staphylococos bovis & *P. albenis*
c) Streptococos bovis & *E. coli*
d) Staphylococcus bovis & *E. coli*

31 Enhancement of lactate utilization can be done by

a) *Propiono bacter* sp.
b) *Rumino bacter* sp.
c) *Rhizopus* sp.
d) Both (a) and (b)

32 Papple shaped abdomen is observed in

a) Ketosis
b) Milk Fever
c) Vagus Indigestion
d) Peri parturient haemoglotrinuria

33 Failure of eructation results in free gas bloat due to inflammatory leisons in the vicinity of vagus nerve is

a) Type-I vagal indigestion
b) Type-II vagal indigestion
c) Type-III vagal indigestion
d) Type-IV vagal indigestion

34 Type II vagal indigestion leads to

a) Cud dropping
b) Failure of omasal transport
c) Abomasal impaction
d) None

35 Type III vagal indigestion is
a) Cud dropping
b) Partial fore stomach obstruction
c) Development of abomasal impaction
d) Reticular obstruction

36 Type IV vagal indigestion is
a) Partial forestomach obstruction
b) Develops in cattle during gestation
c) Related to enlarging uterus shifting the abomasum to more cranial position
d) All of the above

37 Vagal indigestion results in
a) Hyperchloric, hyperkalemic alkalosis
b) Hypochloric, hypokalemic alkslosis
c) Hypochloric, hyperkalemic alkalosis
d) Hyperchloric, hypokalemic alkalosis

38 Common sequare of TRP
a) Acute local peritonitis
b) Acute diffuse peritonitis
c) Both (a) and (b)
d) None of the above

39 Bamboo test is used to diagnose
a) Ruminal acidosis
b) Volvulus
c) TRP
d) Left side displacement of abomasum

40 Protrusion of reticulum and rumen through a rupture of diaphragram
a) Diaphragmatic tension
b) Reticular hernia
c) Diaphragmatic hernia
d) Both (a) and (b)

41 Diaphragmatic hernia is common in
a) Cattle
b) Buffalo
c) Both (a) and (b)
d) Sheep and Goats

42 L-shaped rumen on rectal examination is an indication of
a) Hoflund syndrome
b) TRP
c) TP (Traumatic pericarditis)
d) Paralyticileus

43 D-lactic acidosis in ruminants results in

a) Exudative diarrhoea b) Secretory diarrhoea

c) Osmotic diarrhoea d) Mobility dependent diarrhoea

44 Diarrhoea is generally associated with

a) Alkalosis b) Acidosis

c) Mild alkalosis d) None of the above

45 Vomition is generally associated with

a) Alkalosis b) Severe Acidosis

c) Neither of the above d) Eiher of above

Answer Key

1	b	**2**	d	**3**	c	**4**	a	**5**	b	**6**	b	**7**	c	**8**	d	**9**	b	**10**	b
11	d	**12**	b	**13**	c	**14**	b	**15**	c	**16**	b	**17**	c	**18**	d	**19**	d	**20**	d
21	d	**22**	c	**23**	d	**24**	c	**25**	d	**26**	d	**27**	b	**28**	b	**29**	c	**30**	c
31	a	**32**	c	**33**	a	**34**	b	**35**	c	**36**	d	**37**	b	**38**	c	**39**	c	**40**	c
41	b	**42**	a	**43**	c	**44**	b	**45**	a										

7

Affections of Peritoneum Pancreas and Liver

1 Inflammation of peritonium is called

a) Peronitis
b) Peritonitis
c) Laminitis
d) Oophonitis

2 Blood picture in peritonitis shows

a) Immature neutrophil shift to right
b) Mature neutrophil (shift to left)
c) Immature neutrophil (A degenerative shift to left)
d) None of the above

3 Yellowness of skin and visible mucous membrane (sclera and vaginal mucous), hyper bilirubinemia is called as

a) Icterus
b) Jundice
c) Sclerosis
d) Both (a) and (b)

4 Increased unconjugated bilirubin in serum is seen in

a) Toxic jaundice
b) Prehepatic jundice
c) Posthepatic jaundice
d) Both (b) and (c)

5 The liver function tests are

a) Bromsulthalein charance test
b) Tokata-arotrat
c) Urea tolerance test
d) All of the above

6 Experimentally, which of the followings causes pancreatitis by stimulation

a) Snake venom
b) Scorpion venom
c) Black widow spider venom
d) None of the above

7 Peculiar “prayer position” in dog is observed in

a) Hepatitis
b) Pancreatitis
c) Prochitis
d) Renal ischemia

8 Which breed of dog is more susceptible to exocrine pancreatic insufficiency

a) Doberman b) Spitchz

c) German Shepherd d) Labrador

9 Cherry crandall method is used for estimation of

a) Urine amylase b) Serum lipase

c) Serum alkaline phosphatase d) Serum Calcium

10 BT–PABA Absorption Test is used to diagnose

a) Endocrine pancreatic insufficiency in dogs

b) Exocrine pancreatic insufficiencyin dogs

c) Both of the above

d) None of the above

11 Faeces containing excessive fat is called

a) Amylorrhea b) Creatorrhoea

c) Leptorrhea d) Steatorrhoea

12 Juvenile diabetes is

a) IDDM (Insuline dependent diabetes mellitus)

b) Type-I diabetes

c) Young animals suffer from this type diabetes

d) All of the above

13 Vanden Bergh Test for obstructive jundice is

a) Negative b) Direct positive

c) Biphasic positive d) Indirect positive

14 Color of faeces in post hepatic jundice is

a) Light yellow b) Normal

c) Clay colored d) Greenish yellow

15 In liver disease, Photosensitisation occurs due to accumulation of

a) Phylloerythrin b) Phyllocyanin

c) Xanthophyll d) None of the above

Answer Key

1 b **2** c **3** d **4** b **5** d **6** b **7** b **8** c **9** b **10** b

11 d **12** d **13** b **14** c **15** a

8

Diseases of Cardiovascular System

1. Inflammation of pericardium or pericardial sac is known as
   a) Endocarditis b) Pericarditis
   c) Myocarditis d) Epicarditis
2 On ascultation pericarditis reveals
   a) Muffled heart sound b) Mumming sound
   c) Splashing & gurgling sound d) All of the above
3 Electrocardiography in case of pericarditis reveals
   a) Hydrothorax
   b) Sinus tachycarditis with right sided heart failure
   c) Diminished QRS amplitude
   d) All of the above
4 Fungus causing myocarditis
   a) *Cryptococcus neoformans* b) *Aspergillus flavus*
   c) Trichophyton d) All of the above
5 Tigered heart disease is found in
   a) RP (Rinderpaste) b) RVF
   c) FMD d) PPR
6 Lining of the heart as well as valves within it are affected in
   a) Pericarditis b) Endocarditis
   c) Myocarditis d) None of the above
7 Electrocardiography findings in case of endocarditis
   a) Sinus tachycardia
   b) Ectopic foci
   c) Decreased QRS amplitude in a base apex lead
   d) All of the above

8 Edema of lungs found in

a) Left sided heart failure b) Right sided heart failure

c) Both sided heart failure d) None of the above

9 Congestion of the anterior and posteri or venacava and vein draining blood from the systemic circulation to more larger venous is evident in

a) Left sided CHF b) Right sided CHF

c) Pulmonary congestion d) All of the above

10 Anasarca is characteristically limited to

a) Dorsal surface of body, neck, jaw

b) Lateral surface of body, neck, jaw

c) Ventral surface of body, neck, jaw

d) Both (a) and (b)

11 Digoxin should be given preferably in CHF in ruminants

a) I/V b) I/M

c) Orally d) All

12 In case of acute heart failure, auscultation reveals

a) Cardiac resonance b) Cardiac murmur

c) Cardiac flutter d) Thumping

13 __________ is a cause of Acute Heart Failure death in low

a) Pericarditis b) Endocarditis

c) hypoxia d) Endocarditis

14 Abnormal position of heart outside thoracic cavity

a) Ectopic heart b) Cardiac misplasia

c) Hypoxia d) Cardiomegaly

15 In patent foramen ovale (PFO), a flap like opening allows a shunt form

a) Left to Right atrium b) Right to left atrium

c) Upward to downward d) None of the above

16 VSD (Ventricular septal defect) there is shunting of blood from

a) Right to left ventricle b) Left to right ventricle

c) Upward to downward d) None

17 Failure of closure of ductus arteriosus following birth, PDA (Patent ductus Arteriosus) is a common defect of

a) Horses b) Sheep

c) Goat d) Cattle

18 Fibroclastosis in endocardium is observed in

a) Calves & Lambs b) Calves & Kids

c) Calves & Pig d) Foal and Calves

19 Tetralogy of fallot consists of

a) VSD b) Pulmonary stenosis

c) Dextral position of aorta d) All of the above

20 Bruits is

a) Myocardial rub b) Pulmonary stenosis

c) Dextral position of aorta d) All of the above

Answer Key

1	b	**2**	d	**3**	d	**4**	a	**5**	c	**6**	b	**7**	d	**8**	a	**9**	b	**10**	c
11	a	**12**	b	**13**	b	**14**	a	**15**	b	**16**	b	**17**	a	**18**	c	**19**	d	**20**	b

9

Diseases of Blood & Blood Forming Organs

1 Major haematopoetic organ in adults is

a) Spleen b) Liver

c) Bone marrow d) Kidney

2 _____ in the blood play important role in production of platelets

a) Rubricyte b) Microkaryocytes

c) Reticulocyte d) Megakaryocytes

3 Phenothiazine and chronic copper poisoning leads to

a) Haemorrhagic anemia b) Myeloblastic anemia

c) Haemolytic anemia d) Both (b) and (c)

4 Depression of erythropoesis occurs (crythropoiesis) in

a) Haemorrhagic anemia b) Myeloblastic anemia

c) Haemolytic anemia d) None of the above

5 Transfusion of blood is required when PCV%

a) 12 to 20% b) <12%

c) 12% d) 20 to 24%

6 Which of the following is a altered platelet function (Thrombocytopathies hereditary?

a) Canine thromboplastic disease b) Von-willebrands disease

c) Myeloproliferative disease d) None of the above

7 Ehrlichiosis in dog is associated with

a) Eosinophillia b) Neutrophillia

c) Thrmbocytopenia d) Basophilia

8 Anemia associated with poor oxygenation of blood

a) Anaemic hypoxia b) Anoxic hypoxia

c) Stagnant hypoxia d) None of the above

9 Radiation and Radiomimetic drugs produce

a) Leukopenia b) Leukocytosis

c) Lymphocytosis d) Monocytosis

10 A regenerative left shift is characterized by

a) Absolute increase in neutrophills

b) Appearance of mature neutrophil

c) Appearance of immature neutrophill

d) Both (a) and (c)

11 Inability of bone marrow to produce mature cells in response to infections indicates

a) Degenerative left shift b) Degenerative right shift

c) Regenerative left shift d) Regenerative right shift

12 Localised infections like traumatic peritonitis is manifested by

a) 70 to 80 % neutrophils in circulation with matured neutrophil

b) 90 to 95% neutrophils in circulation with large no.of immature neutrophils

c) 90 to 95 % neutrophills in circulation and large no. of mature neutrophil

d) 70 to 80% neutrophils in circulation with large no. of immature neutrophills

13 CFU-GM (Colony forming granulocyte and monocyte) is responsible for production of

a) Neutrophil b) Basophil

c) Monocyte d) Both (a) and (b)

14 Which of the following statements is correct

a) Chronic granulocytopathy syndrome is common in Irrish setter

b) Chronifrancatocy to pathy syndrome is common in young animal

c) Geriatric dogs have monocytosis

d) All of the above

15 Hodgkin lymphoma is a form of cancer involving

a) Monocytosis b) Eosinophilia

c) Basophilia d) Both (a) and (b)

16 Hyper lipoproteinemia is associated with

a) Basophilia b) Eosionophellia

c) Neutrophilia d) Monocytosis

17 Long "ribbon –like" nucleus is found in

a) Eosinophil b) Basophil

c) Neutrophil d) Lymphocyte

18 In Hog cholera

a) There is panleukopenia in early stage

b) There is leukocytosis in early stages

c) There is neutrophilia in early stages

d) None of the above

19 Folic acid defreeency is associated with

a) Monocytic anemia b) Mrrocytic hypochromic anaemia

c) Macrocytic anemia d) Microcytic anaemia

20 Steroid therapy shows

a) Eosino cosinopenia b) Eosinophilia

c) Basophilia d) Lymphocytosis

Answer Key

1	c	**2**	d	**3**	c	**4**	c	**5**	b	**6**	d	**7**	c	**8**	b	**9**	a	**10**	d
11	a	**12**	b	**13**	d	**14**	d	**15**	d	**16**	a	**17**	b	**18**	a	**19**	c	**20**	a

10

Diseases of Respiratory System

1 Defective oxygenation of blood in pulmonary circulation

a) Anaemic anoxia b) Stagnant anoxia

c) Anoxic anoxia d) Histotoxic anoxia

2 Basic defect in congestive heart failure

a) Anaemic anoxia b) Stagnant anoxia

c) Anoxic anoxia d) Histotoxic anoxia

3 Deficiency of haemoglobin per unit volume of blood reducing oxygen carrying capacity of blood causes

a) Anaemic anoxia b) Stagnant anoxia

c) Anoxic anoxia d) Histotoxic anoxia

4 Cyanide poisoning causes

a) Histotoxic anoxia b) Stagnant anoxia

c) Anoxic anoxia d) Anaemic anoxia

5 Respiratory centre is located in

a) Cerebrum b) Medulla

c) Cerebellum d) None of the above

6 Hypercapnea and anoxia are marked in

a) Paralytic respiratory failure b) Dyspnoeic respiratory failure

c) Asphyxial respiratory failure d) Tachypnoeic respiratory failure

7 Poisoning with respiratorycentre depressants causes

a) Paralytic respiratory failure b) Dyspnoeic respiratory failure

c) Asphyxial respiratory failure d) Both (b) and (c)

8 In hyperthermia there is

a) Dull respiratory failure b) Dyspnoeri respiratory failure

c) Asphyxial respiratory failure d) Tachypnoic respiratory failure

9 Explosive expiration of air from lungs is called

a) Cough b) Wheeze

c) Snore d) Snidor

10 Sudden noisy expiration through nasal cavities caused reflexly by nasal mucosa irritation

a) Coughing b) Sneezing

c) Wheeze d) Snore

11 High pitched sound produced by air coming through narrow lumen is termed as

a) Cough b) Snore

c) Wheeze d) Stertor

12 An inspiratory stenotic sound originating from reduction in the calliber of larynx is called

a) Snore b) Stertor

c) Snidor d) Wheeze

13 Deep guttural sound on inspiration originating from vibration of pharyngeal mucosa is termed as

a) Snore b) Stertor

c) Snidor d) Wheeze

14 Cyanosis is absent in

a) Histotoxic anoxia b) Anoxic anoxia

c) Stagnant anoxia d) Anaemic anoxia

15 Foul smelling nasal discharge is

a) Halitosis b) Plurosis

c) Ozera d) None of the above

16 A copious bilateral nasal discharge suggests

a) Allergic rhinitis b) Bacterial rhinitis

c) Both (a) and (b) d) None of the above

17 Coughing/ Spitting of blood from lungs is called

a) Epistaxis b) Haemoptysis

c) Haemorhoids d) Haematochezia

18 Nose bleeding is termed as

a) Epistaxis b) Haemoptysis

c) Haemotochezia d) Melena

19 The site for insertion of needle for thoracocentesis

a) 4th to 5th intercostal space b) 5th to 6th intercostal space
c) 9th to 10th intercostal space d) 6th to7^{th} intercostal space

20 For lungs tissue therapy, tissue is taken from trocar and canula at

a) 4th to 5th intercostal space b) 6th to 7th intercostal space
c) 8th to 9th intercostal space d) 5th to 6th intercostal space

21 Spirography is used

a) To boost for vital capacity of lungs b) Detect residual volumes
c) Detect respiratory volume d) All of the above

22 Estimation of CO_2 content of expired air is done by

a) Capnography b) Oxygraphy
c) Carbography d) Both (a) and (b)

23 Chronic rhinitis condition is prevalent in

a) Glander in horse b) Rhinosporidiosis
c) Schistosoma nasalis in cattle d) All of the above

24 Inhalation of chemical vapour like ammonia, chlorine, sulphate etc. leads to

a) Chronic rhinitis b) Acute rhinitis
c) Both d) None of the above

25 Dogs having dry, harsh and hacking type of cough upon exposure to cold, dust, excitement is suflening from

a) Acute rhinitis b) Acute laryngitis
c) Chronic laryngitis d) Chronr rhinitis

26 Ronchi is

a) Due to narrowing of lumen b) Also called as Dry Rales
c) Due to wide opening of bronchi d) Both (a) and (b)

27 Inflammation of lung parenchyma usually accompanied with inflammation of bronchiole with pleura is known as

a) Bronchitis b) Pneumonia
c) Pleuritis d) Tracheitis

28 Fungus causing pneumonia

a) Histoplasmosis b) *Aspergillus fumigatus*
c) Blastomycosis d) All of the above

29 Bacterial agents causing pneumonia in pig

a) Pasteurella b) Haemophilus

c) Salmonella d) All of the above

30 Bacteria causing pnermonia by haematogenous route

a) *Corynebacterium pyogens* b) *Pasteurella* sp.

c) TB (*Mycobacterium tuberculosis*) d) *Staphylococous* sp.

31 In early stage of bacterial pneumonia

a) Ventricular murmur is prominent b) Transient sound is prominent

c) Dry rales are observed d) Both (b) and (c)

32 Dry unproductive cough, hacking nature is seen in

a) Bacterial pneumonia b) Parasitic pneumonia

c) Bronchiothorax d) Cardiothorax

33 Accumulation of air in pleural space is called

a) Pneumothorax b) Sangus pleura

c) Haemothorax d) Haemorrhagic thorax

34 Accumulation of blood in pleural sac

a) Pneumothorax b) Sangus pleura

c) Haemothorax d) Haemorrhagic thorax

35 Hydrothorax is

a) Accumulation of exudates in thoracic cavity

b) Accumulation of transudate in thoracic cavity

c) Accumulation of blood in thoracic cavity

d) Accumulation of air in thoracic cavity

Answer Key

1	c	**2**	b	**3**	a	**4**	a	**5**	b	**6**	c	**7**	a	**8**	d	**9**	a	**10**	b
11	c	**12**	c	**13**	d	**14**	d	**15**	c	**16**	c	**17**	b	**18**	a	**19**	d	**20**	c
21	d	**22**	a	**23**	d	**24**	b	**25**	c	**26**	d	**27**	b	**28**	d	**29**	d	**30**	c
31	a	**32**	c	**33**	a	**34**	c	**35**	b										

11

Diseases of Urinary System

1 Homeostasis in kidney is generally maintained by

a) Glomerulus b) Renal tubules

c) Both (a) and (b) d) None of the above

2 Excretion of metabolic end products is controlled by

a) Glomerulus b) Renal tubules

c) Renal crust d) None of the above

3 Blood in urine is called

a) Haemoglobinuria b) Haematuria

c) Pyouria d) Myoglobinuria

4 Azoturia in horses indicates

a) Myoglobin in urine b) Dark brown urine

c) Not very high plasma level of myoglobin d) All of the above

5 Enterotoxemia due to *Clostridium perfringe* soccurs in association with

a) Proteinuria b) Crystalluria

c) Glycosuria d) Pyouria

6 In diabetes mellitus, there is

a) Only glycousuria b) Glycosuria with ketourea

c) Only ketouria d) Glycous uria with crystalluria

7 Reduction in daily output of urine is called

a) Dysuria b) Oliguria

c) Anuria d) Polyuria

8 Increase in volume of urine production

a) Pyouria b) Polyuria

c) Anuria d) Oliguria

9 Complete absence of urine flow

a) Anuria b) Starvation in cattle

c) Pyuria d) Oligouria

10 Common findings of ketouria in ruminants occurs in

a) Ketonemia in cattle b) Starvation in cattle

c) Pregnancy toxemia d) All of the above

11 Painful or difficult urination is called

a) Azoturia b) Dysuria

c) Oliguria d) Polyuria

12 Chronic renal disease is usually manifested by

a) Polyuria b) Oligouria

c) Anuria d) None of the above

13 Clinical signs of uremia are

a) Anuria b) Oliguria

c) Myoglobinuria d) Both (a) and (b)

14 The most common cause of acute renal failure is

a) Nephrosis b) Ureteritis

c) Cystitis d) All of the above

15 What is an early indication of damage to renal parenchyma

a) Ketouria b) Polyuria

c) Proteinuria d) Myoglobinuria

16 Proliferative glomerulonephritis is relatively common cause of

a) Acute renal failure in horse b) Peracute renal failure in horse

c) Chronic renal failure in horse d) Subclinical renal failure in horse

17 System that plays major role in pathogenesis of glomerular lesion

a) Cardiovascular system b) Digestive system

c) Immune system d) Reproductive system

18 BUN (Blood Urea Nitrogen) is increased with hypophosphatemia and hypocalcemia in

a) Pyelonephritis b) Glomerulonephritis

c) Interstitial nephritis d) Cystitis

19 In pigs, diffused interstitial nephritis is observed in

a) Leptospirosis b) Listeriosis

c) Swine erysipelas d) None of the above

20 Ascending infection from lower urinary tract characterised by pyuria, suppurative nephritis, cystitis and ureterit is

a) Interstitial nephritis b) Glomerular nephritis

c) Pyelonephritis d) Renal ischemia

21 Specific pyolonephritis in cattle is caused by

a) Eubacterium iris b) *Corynebacterium renale*

c) Leptospira sp. d) *E. coli*

22 Specific pyelonephritis in pigs is caused by

a) *Eubacterium iris* b) Leptospirosis

c) *E. coli* d) Listeriosis

23 Inflammation of urinary bladder is called

a) Nephritis b) Cystitis

c) Uteritis d) endometritis

24 Urolithiasis is an important clinical disease of

a) Castrated male ruminants b) Uncastrated male ruminants

c) Both (a) and (b) d) None of the above

25 Surgical treatment for urolithiasis

a) Urethral removal b) Urethrostomy

c) Relieving of bladder pressure d) Both (b) and (c)

Answer Key

1 b	**2** a	**3** b	**4** d	**5** c	**6** b	**7** b	**8** b	**9** a	**10** d
11 b	**12** a	**13** d	**14** a	**15** c	**16** c	**17** c	**18** b	**19** a	**20** c
21 b	**22** a	**23** b	**24** a	**25** d					

12

Diseases of Lymphatic System

1 Lymphnodes are found in every part of the body except

a) Digestive system b) Respiratory system

c) Cardiovascular system d) Central nervous system

2 Major organs of lymphatic system are

a) Spleen b) Thymus

c) Bone marrow d) All of the above

3 Most of the lymphnodes and lymphatic tissues are located in and around

a) Gastrointestinal tract b) Respiratory tract

c) Reproductive tract d) Urinary tract

4 Enlargement of lymph nodes is called

a) Lymphangitis b) Lymphoma

c) Lymphadanepathy d) None

5 Caseous lymphadenitis is caused by

a) *Streptococcus pyogens* b) *Staphylococous aureus*

c) *Burkholderia pseudomollei* d) *Corynebacterium pseudotuberculosis*

6 Caseous lymphadenitis is a _________ disease

a) Acute b) Chronic

c) Subacute d) Peracute

7 Transmission of caseous lymphadenitis causing bacteria takes place by

a) Contaminated food, bedding and equipments

b) Open skin wound

c) Mucous membrane of mouth and lungs

d) All of the above

8 Caseous lymphadenatis is manifested by

a) Abscesses in lymph nodes b) Closed and swollen abscess

c) Open draining sores d) All of the above

9 Epizootic lymphangitis is also known as

a) Pseudo farcy b) Equine histoplasmosis

c) Pseudo glanders d) All of the above

10 Equine histoplasmosis is presented clinically as

a) Pulmonary form b) Pyogranulomotous form

c) Occular form d) All of the above

11 Epizootic lymphangitis spreads through

a) Contaminated food b) Flies and ticks

c) Open skin wound d) All of the above

12 Lymphosarcoma in adult cattle is seen in the age group

a) 3-6 years b) 5-8 years

c) 2-3 years d) 10-12 years

13 Major source of Bovine leukemia virus infection is

a) Blood b) Colostrum

c) Milk d) All of the above

14 Bovine leukemia virus may also affect

a) Sheep b) Pig

c) Goat d) Horses

15 Which of the following statements false regarding Bovine leukemia virus associated Lymphosarcoma

a) Only 2-5% positive for BLV develop lymphosarcoma

b) Prevalance of disease is influenced by susceptibility of animals due to genetic and managemental factors

c) Natural service or artificial insemination is one of the major sources of infection

d) Sheep are much more susceptible to infection than cows

16 Nucleus to cytoplasmic ratio in lymphosarcoma is

a) Higher b) Does not change

c) Lower d) Changes under certain conditions

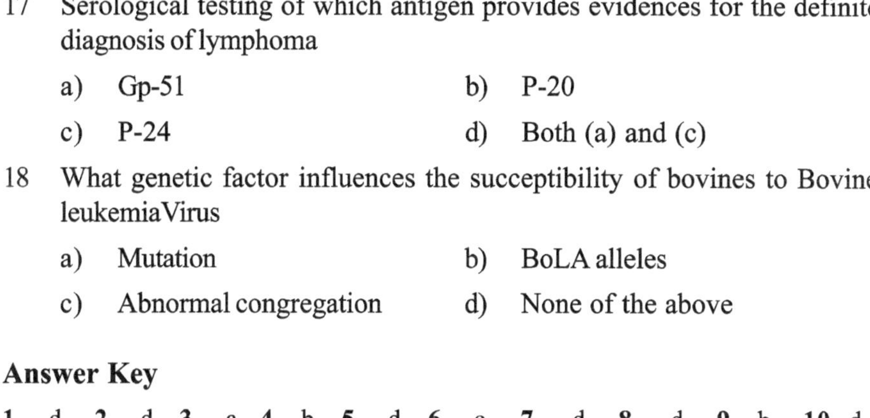

17 Serological testing of which antigen provides evidences for the definite diagnosis of lymphoma

a) Gp-51 b) P-20

c) P-24 d) Both (a) and (c)

18 What genetic factor influences the succeptibility of bovines to Bovine leukemiaVirus

a) Mutation b) BoLA alleles

c) Abnormal congregation d) None of the above

Answer Key

1 d **2** d **3** a **4** b **5** d **6** c **7** d **8** d **9** b **10** d

11 d **12** d **13** a **14** d **15** a **16** c **17** d **18** d

13

Diseases of Conjunctiva Skin and External Ear

1 Condition characterised by bran - like scales on skin surfaces is called
   a) Pustule   b) Parakeratosis
   c) Erythema   d) Pityriasis

2 Causes for pityriasis/dandruff includes
   a) Dietary deficiency of Vitamin A and B complex
   b) Flea, Lice and mange infestation
   c) Iodine poisoning
   d) All of the above

3 Incomplete keratinisation of the epithellial cells is called
   a) Parakeratosis   b) Pachyderma
   c) Hyperkeratosis   d) Urticaria

4 Dietary deficiency of which minerals cause parakeratosis
   a) Mn   b) Zn & Se
   c) Ca & P   d) Cu

5 Parakeratosis affects Which layer of epidermis is affected in parakeratosis?
   a) Stratum granulosum   b) Stratum basale
   c) Stratum corneum   d) Both (a) and (b)

6 Treatment of dandruff includes
   a) Salicylic acid containing lotion
   b) Alcoholic solution
   c) Thorough washing with keratolytic shampoo
   d) All of the above

7 Excessive keratinisation of the epithelial cells is called
   a) Parakeratosis   b) Dermatitis
   c) Hyperkeratosis   d) Pityriasis

8 Etiology of hyperkeratosis includes

a) Poisoning with napthaline b) Inherited congenital ichthyosis

c) Chronic arsenic poisoning d) All of the above

9 Clinical findings of hyperkeratosis

a) Skin becomes thicker and corrugated

b) Dry, scaly and hairless external surface

c) Development of fissures

d) All of the above

10 Which skin layer is affected in pachyderma?

a) Stratum granulosum b) Stratum spinosum

c) Stratum basale d) All the layers

11 Superficial eruptions of thin-walled small vesicles surrounded by a zone of erythema is called

a) Impetigo b) Acne

c) Pustule d) Scab

12 In animals, impetigo gets infected secondarily by

a) *Staphylococous* sp. b) *Corynobacterium* sp.

c) *Streptococous* sp. d) None of the above

13 Allergic condition characterised by appearance of wheals on skin is called as

a) Impetigo b) Urticaria

c) Erythema d) Boils

14 Urticaria lesions have following characterstics except

a) Large in number and develop rapidly b) Elevated with flat top

c) Always itching d) Without exudates

15 Drug of choice for urticaria may be

a) Antihistamines b) Cooling astringent lotion

c) Epinephrine d) All of the above

16 Dermatitis is defined as inflammation of

a) Epidermis b) Dermis

c) Both Dermis and Epidermis d) Subcutaneous tissue

17 Etiology of dermatitis includes

a) Fungal infection
b) Photosensitivity
c) Parasitic infection
d) All of the above

18 Complications of dermatitis include

a) Cellulitis
b) Toxaemia
c) Septicemia
d) All of the above

19 Inflammation of the conjunctiva and the layers below is called

a) Conjuctivities
b) keratoconjunctivitis
c) Blepharitis
d) All of the above

20 Clinical signs that may be seen in conjuctivitis

a) Blepharospasm
b) Vascularisation of cornea
c) Watery tears followed by occular discharge with pus
d) All of the above

21 Solid skin like masses of tissue that usually adhere to the anterior surface of eye causing irritation

a) Stye
b) Dermoid cyst
c) Dentigerous cyst
d) None of the above

22 Otitis externa is

a) Inflammation of external ear canal
b) Painful ear pinna
c) Inflammation of the whole ear
d) Inflammation of middle ear canna

23 Common cause of otitis externa in cattle is

a) Thelazia species
b) Strongylids
c) Rhabditis boxi?
d) Arthropod parasite

24 Clinical signs of otitis externa in cattle may be

a) Frequent head shaking
b) Alopecia below both the ear
c) Pain while swallowing
d) All of the above

Answer Key

1 d **2** d **3** a **4** c **5** b **6** d **7** b **8** d **9** d **10** c

11 a **12** a **13** c **14** c **15** d **16** c **17** d **18** d **19** c **20** d

21 c **22** a **23** b **24** d

14

Diseases of Musculoskeletal System

1 The clinical manifestations of disease of muscle, bones and joints are generally characterised by

a) Lameness b) Failure of support to stand

c) Incoordination of movement d) All of the above

2 Degenerative disease of bones is called as

a) Osteomyelitis b) Osteodystrophy

c) Arthropathy d) Osteomalacia

3 Degenerative disease of muscles

a) Myositis b) Myositis ossificans

c) Myopathy d) Myosthenia

4 Treatment of myositis includes

a) Use of antimicrobials b) Use of anti-inflammatory drug

c) Both (a) and (b) d) Fomentation

5 Skeletal muscle asthenia is called as

a) Ischemia b) Myosthenia

c) Muscular dystrophy d) Marasmus

6 Distinctive features of Myasthenia

a) Paresis b) Paralysis

c) Incoordination d) All of the above

7 Myopathy is pathologically characterised by

a) Fibrinous degenaration b) Mucinous degeneration

c) Hyaline degeneration d) Hydropic degenaration

8 In myopathy, which of the following muscle enzymes are elevated

a) CPK b) SGOT

c) SGPT and BUN d) Both (a) and (b)

9 Which of the following is a common finding in myopathy

a) Haemoglobinuria b) Myoglobinuria

c) Hematuria d) Crystalluria

10 Enzootic nutritional muscular distrophy is caused due to deficiency of

a) Vitamin-A b) Vitamin-D

c) Vitamin-E d) Vitamin-B1

11 Congenital degenerative myopathy occuring in new born calves is due to infection by

a) Akabane Virus b) Orbivirus

c) Bluetongue Virus d) Birna virus

12 Increase in CPK level indicates degeneration of

a) Skeletal muscles only

b) Myocardial muscle only

c) Both myocardial and skeletal muscles

d) Excess intake of protein through diet

13 In myopathy, affected areas of skeletal muscle have an appearance like

a) Proud flesh b) Fish flesh

c) Granulating tissue d) None of the above

14 Nutritional muscular dystrophy can be treated by administration of

a) Vitamin A, D & E b) Vitamin D3 and Calcium

c) Vitamin B and C d) Vitamin E and Selenium

15 To prevent myoglobinuric nephrosis in cases of myopathy

a) Intravenous fluid therapy should be given

b) High protein diet should be given

c) Provision of palatable nutritious food is indicated

d) Both (a) and (c)

16 Myositis refers to

a) Non-inflammatory degeneration of muscle

b) Inflammatory condition of muscle

c) Excessive growth of muscular tissue

d) All of the above

17 Chronic lead poisoning causes
   a) Osteoporosis in lambs and foals
   b) Osteomalacia in adult horses
   c) Both of the above
   d) None of the above

18 In osteodystrophy, the level of serum alkaline phosphatase is
   a) Decreased
   b) Elevated
   c) Not affected
   d) Increases in acute cases and decreases in chronic cases

19 Bacteria can reach into bone by
   a) Hematogenous
   b) Exterior from an adjacent route focus of infection
   c) By direct inoculation via trauma or surgery
   d) All of the above

20 Secondary osteoarthropathy is
   a) Normal ageing process
   b) Initiated by injuries or congenital, conformational defects
   c) Disturbances in normal differentiation of cells in growing cartilages
   d) All of the above

21 Osteochondrosis is
   a) Degeneration and erosion of articular cartilage
   b) Hypertrophy of bone surrounding articular cartilage
   c) Disturbances in normal differentiation of cells in growing cartilage
   d) All of the above

22 In neonates, arthritis is accompanied by
   a) Omphalophlebitis   b) Swelling of lymphnodes
   c) Inguinal hernia   d) None of the above

23 In arthritis most commonly involved joint is/are
   a) Hock   b) Stifle
   c) Knee   d) All of the above

24 Which of the following is a non-inflammatory condition of bone

a) Osteochondrosis b) Arthritis

c) Osteomyelitis d) None of the above

Answer Key

1	d	**2**	b	**3**	c	**4**	c	**5**	b	**6**	d	**7**	c	**8**	d	**9**	b	**10**	c
11	a	**12**	c	**13**	b	**14**	d	**15**	d	**16**	b	**17**	a	**18**	b	**19**	d	**20**	b
21	c	**22**	a	**23**	d	**24**	a												

15

Diseases of Nervous System

1 Inflammation of meninges and spinal cord along with brain is called

a) Encephalomyelitis
b) Encephalitis
c) Meningitis
d) Meningoencephalitis

2 Verminous encephalitis in horses is caused by

a) Equine infectious anemia
b) *Strongylus vulgaris*
c) *Listeria monocytogenes*
d) Migration of *Oestrus ovius*

3 Which of the following is the degenerative disease of CNS characterised by softening of brain

a) Encephalitis
b) Encephalomyletis
c) Both (a) and (b)
d) Encephalomalacia

4 Hepatic encephalopathy in advanced liver disease occurs due to

a) Low level of ammonia in blood
b) High level of ammonia in blood
c) Low level of glucose in blood
d) High level of bilirubin

5 In ruminants cause of encephalomalacia is

a) Bovine sponge form encephalopathy
b) Infection with *Clostridium perfringen* type D
c) Thermotoxicity
d) Both (a) and (c)

6 Cerebral edema can be treated with intravenous adminstration of

a) Mannitol
b) Furosemide
c) Spironolactone
d) All of the above

7 Feeding of moldy corn infected with Fusarium moniliforme in horses leads to

a) Arthritis
b) Encephalomalacia
c) Encephalitis
d) Spondylitis

8 Pathogens responsible for brain edema is/are

a) *Actinobacillus mallei* b) *Streptococcus zooepidemicus*

c) *Staphylococcus aureus* d) All of the above

9 Coenurosis is caused by invasion of brain and spinal cord by

a) Larvae of *Oestrus ovis*

b) Intermediate stage of *Tenia multiceps*

c) Intermediate stage *Coenurus cerebralis*

d) Both (b) and (c)

10 Causes of meningitis in horses

a) *Cryptococcus neoformans* b) *Listeria* sp.

c) *Histophilus somni* d) Tuberculosis

11 Clinical signs of meningitis is produced by irritation of

a) CNS b) PNS

c) Both (a) and (b) d) None of the above

12 Examination of CSF in meningitis reveals

a) Low protein concentration b) High protein concentration

c) Low cell count d) No changes

13 Neuropsy finding in meningitis shows

a) Haermorrhages b) Thick binding of meningitis

c) Inflammation of meningus d) All of the above

14 Condition that results from a sudden and uncontrolled electric discharge of neurons in the cerebral cortex is

a) Seizure b) Encephalitis

c) Mania d) All of the above

15 The term used for generalised seizures with a specific EEG pattern is

a) Grand mal b) Petit mal

c) Cluster ceizures d) None of the above

16 A serial of seizures within a short period of time, in a dog regaining consciousness between seizures is termed as

a) Grand Mal b) Encephalitis

c) Mania d) None of the above

17 Rapidly repeating seizures with no period of consciousness between them

a) Grand Mal b) Status epileptious

c) Petit mMal d) Clusters seizures

18 First phase of seizure lasts for

a) 60 sec b) 10-30 sec

c) 130 sec d) More than a minute

19 During seizure, the animal has uncons ciousness, rigidity and extends the legs in

a) Toxic phase b) Two-Chronic phase

c) Classic Phase d) None of the above

20 In chronic phase of seizure

a) Animals legs make running or paddling movements

b) May urinate and defecate

c) Mouth makes chewing motions

d) All of the above

Answer Key

1	a	**2**	c	**3**	d	**4**	c	**5**	d	**6**	a	**7**	c	**8**	d	**9**	d	**10**	a
11	c	**12**	c	**13**	d	**14**	a	**15**	c	**16**	b	**17**	c	**18**	c	**19**	a	**20**	d

16

Metabolic Diseases

1 Metabolic profile test to know the nutritional status of a dairy animal, by assessing the blood used components

a) Complete profile test b) Metabolic profile test

c) Compton metabolic profile test d) Dairy animal metabolism test

2 Milk fever is also known as

a) Parturient paresis b) Calving paralysis

c) Parturient apoplexy d) All of the above

3 Milk fever occurs when the level of ionised calcium in blood is below

a) 2-3 mg/dl b) 10 mg/dl

c) 5-6 mg/dl d) 14 mg/dl

4 Lateral bending of head towards flank is seen in which stage of milk fever

a) Stage of excitement b) Stage of lateral recumbency

c) Stage of sternal recumbency d) All the stages

5 Eclampsia in bitch is mostly clear during

a) Late gestation b) 1-2 months after whelping

c) 3 weeks after whelping d) All of the above

6 Eclampsia occurs due to

a) Hypercalcemia b) Hypocalcemia

c) Hypophosphatemia d) Hypokalemia

7 Hypocalcemia in mare causes

a) Grass tetany b) Wheat pasture tetany

c) Lactation tetany d) None of the above

8 Downers cow syndrome is a complication of

a) Hypocalcemia b) Hypercalcemia

c) Hyponatremia d) Hypermagnesemia

9 "Creeper Cows" with "frog leg posture" are associated with

a) Milk fever
b) Ketosis
c) Downer's Cow syndrome
d) Hypomagnesemia

10 Complication of Downer's Cow syndrome is

a) Cessation of urination
b) Decubitus ulcer
c) Reduced appetite
d) All of the above

11 CPK levels with experimental Downer Cow increase

a) Immediately when recumbent
b) Within 12 to 24 hours
c) Within 6 hours
d) After 9 hours

12 Ketosis is characterised by

a) Hypoglycemia
b) Ketolactia
c) Ketonemia
d) All of the above

13 The type of ketosis seen when the dairy animal is fed with silage with excess amount of butarate

a) Primary ketosis
b) Secondary ketosis
c) Alimentary ketosis
d) None of the above

14 Ketosis due to deficiency of propionate protein is called as

a) Primary ketosis
b) Starvation ketosis
c) Predustine ketosis
d) Secondary ketosis

15 Normal level of ketone bodies in milk

a) 3 mg/dl
b) 40 mg/dl
c) 10 mg/dl
d) Nil

16 Nervous form of ketosis must be differentiated from

a) Rabies
b) Lead poisoning
c) Laryngeal paralysis
d) All of the above

17 Compounds helpful in prevention of ketosis that may be given in the diet

a) Magnesium
b) Niacin
c) Sodium propionate
d) All of the above

18 Pregnancy toxemia in Ewes is also known as

a) Ovine ketosis
b) Twin lamb disease
c) Kidney disease
d) All of the above

19 Pregnancy toxemia occurs in the
   a) Last 4th to 6th week before parturition
   b) Mid gestation
   c) Within 24 to 48 hours of parturition
   d) Two weeks after parturition

20 Clinical signs of animal ketosis includes
   a) Muscle tremors b) Star-grazing positions
   c) Tenesmus d) All of the above

21 Grass stagger is a production disease that occurs due to deficiency of
   a) Copper b) Selenium
   c) Magnesium d) All of the above

22 Grass tetany is clinically manifested by
   a) Hyperaesthesia b) Opisthotomus
   c) Consciousness d) All of the above

23 Minimal manifestation of hypomagnesemia tetany is seen when the serum magnesium level is
   a) Below 3 mg/dl b) Below 1 mg/dl
   c) Below 5 mg/dl d) Below 4 mg/dl

24 The following are the factors that decrease bioavailability of magnesium except
   a) High potassium content in diet
   b) Heavy top dressing of fodder with Nitrogen fertilizers
   c) Hot and dry weather
   d) Ingestion of protein -rich diet

25 Hypomagnesemic tetany is clinically manifested in
   a) Acute form b) Sub acute form
   c) Chronic form d) All of the above

26 The normal CSF magnesium level is
   a) 3 mg/dl b) 2 mg/dl
   c) 1 mg/dl d) 4 mg/dl

27 Even after 48 hours of death, which body sample can be analysed for true reflection of magnesium level
   a) Blood b) Vitreous humour
   c) CSF d) None of the above

28 Azoturia is also known as

a) Mon day morning sickness b) Tying-up

c) Paralytic myoglobinuria d) All of the above

29 Azoturia is a disease of

a) Cattle b) Horses

c) Dogs and Cats d) Sheep and Goat

30 Precipitating factor for Azoturia

a) Se toxicity b) Bad weather

c) Deficiency of vit-E and Se d) Protein deficient food

31 Dark brown coloured urine in Azoturia is due to

a) Myoglobin b) Haemoglobin

c) Ruptured RBC d) Increased blood cell count

32 Death in Azoturia may be due to

a) Decubitus septicemia b) Uremia

c) Myoglobinuric nephrosis d) All of the above

33 Serum profile of an animal affected with azoturia

a) Increased CPK b) Increased SGOT

c) Both (a) and (b) d) None of the above

34 Osteodystrophy fibrosa is a disease of

a) Horse b) Sheep and Goat

c) Pig d) All of the above

35 Etiology of osteodystrophy fibrosa includes

a) Excessive serum phosphorous b) Secondary calcium deficiency

c) Chronic interstitial nephritis d) All of the above

36 Clinical signs of osteodystrophy fibrosa include

a) Shifting lamnesses b) Enlargement of facial bones

c) Swelling of joints d) Cadmium toxicity

37 The most common predisposing factor in case of post parturient hemoglobinurea is

a) Hyperphosphataemia b) Hypophosphataemia

c) Selenium deficiency d) Selenium toxicity

38 Phosphorus level in serum in case of post-parturient haemoglobinurea is

a) 0.9 to 1.5 mg/dl b) 0.2 to 0.3 mg/dl
c) 2-3 mg/dl d) 1-2 mg/dl

39 Differential diagnosis of post-parturient haemoglobinuria includes

a) Leptospirosis b) Babesiosis
c) Copper poisoning d) All of the above

40 Hypothyroidism is primarily a disease of

a) Adult dogs b) Obesity and intolerance to cold
c) Lack of libido d) All of the above

41 Recommended dose of levothyroxin in mild to mild to moderate hypothyroidism in dogs is

a) 20μ gm /kg wt b) 50μ gm /kg wt
c) 5μ gm /kg wt d) 10μ gm /kg wt

42 Clinical signs of diabetes mellitus in dogs

a) Polyuria b) Obesity
c) Polydypsia d) All of the above

43 Diabetes insipidus is due to

a) Deficiency in insulin hormone b) Defective response to ADH
c) Increased ADH d) Defective release of angiotensin

Answer Key

1	b	**2**	d	**3**	b	**4**	b	**5**	b	**6**	c	**7**	b	**8**	a	**9**	c	**10**	c
11	c	**12**	d	**13**	c	**14**	b	**15**	a	**16**	d	**17**	d	**18**	d	**19**	a	**20**	d
21	c	**22**	d	**23**	b	**24**	c	**25**	d	**26**	b	**27**	c	**28**	d	**29**	c	**30**	b
31	a	**32**	d	**33**	c	**34**	d	**35**	d	**36**	d	**37**	b	**38**	a	**39**	d	**40**	a
41	a	**42**	d	**43**	c														

17

Nutritional Deficiency Diseases

1 Application of lime reduces plant minerals namely

a) Ca b) Zn

c) Mn d) All of the above

2 Excess Ca in diet interferes with the absorption of

a) Iodine b) Cadmium

c) Lead d) All of the above

3 Vitamin A sparer is

a) Vitamin E b) Vitamin B1

c) Vitamin D d) Vitamin C

4 Storage of copper in the body is reduced by

a) Nitrates and nitrites b) Sulphur

c) Molybdenum d) Both (b) and (c)

5 Predisposing factor for energy deficiency is

a) Poor quality feed b) Inclement weather

c) High producing animal d) All of the above

6 Economic loss due to protein deficiency is

a) Slow growth rate b) Reduced rate production

c) Delayed onset of puberty d) All of the above

7 Protein malnutrition occurs less commonly in

a) Dairy Cattle b) Sheep

c) Goat d) Calf fed with whole cow milk

8 Prevention of protein deficiency can be done by following except

a) Age-appropriate feed

b) Monitoring body condition and nutritional states

c) Regular analysis of feed

d) Providing costly feed

9 Lactation tetany due to magnesium deficiency is a disease of

a) Dog and cat b) Horses

c) Sheep and Goat d) Cattle

10 Most prominent clinical signs in magnesium deficiency are

a) Hyperaesthesia b) Paralysis

c) Uncontrolled pacing d) Brown coloured urine

11 Cobalt deficiency in diet results in deficiency of

a) Molybdenum b) Vitamin B12

c) Calcium d) Zinc

12 Animal most susceptible to cobalt deficiency

a) Horses b) Cows and Lambs

c) Dog d) Both (b) and (c)

13 Clinical signs of cobalt deficiency in sheep includes

a) Retarded growth b) Reduced lambing percent

c) Reduced production d) All of the above

14 Characterstic post-mortem lesion in cobalt deficiency

a) Congested spleen b) Polycystic kidney

c) Greyish liver d) Yellow deposition in liver

15 Lambs from cobalt deficient ewes are

a) Slower to start sucking and therefore have low serum immunoglobulin

b) May suffer from photosensitisation in acute cases

c) Anaemia and emaciation seen in acute cases

d) All of the above

16 When the dietary intake is sufficient but the utilisation of copper by tissue is impaired, it is called

a) Primary deficiency b) Dietary deficiency

c) Secondary deficiency d) Both (a) and (b)

17 Animal susceptible to copper poisoning

a) Goat b) Horses

c) Sheep d) Pig

18 Administration of which of the following minerals may increase copper absorption in sheeps

a) Selenium b) Molybdenum

c) Calcium d) Zinc

19 Copper is important for body as it is

a) Component of ceruloplasmin

b) Deficiency causes diarrrhoea associated with molybdenosis

c) Necessary for formation of myosin

d) All of the above

20 Clinical signs of copper deficiency in cattle are

a) Production loss b) Itching and hair licking

c) Rough hair coat d) All of the above

21 Falling disease is due to

a) Deficiency of copper b) Deficiency of Calcium

c) Energy deficient diet d) Iron deficiency

22 Characterstic features of falling disease

a) Intermittent bellowing b) Instant death after falling

c) Both (a) and (b) d) None of the above

23 Pit score teat is caused by

a) Secondary Copper deficiency b) Molybdenum poisoning

c) Both (a) and (b) d) Primary copper deficiency

24 Copper deficiency in sheep show

a) Depigmentation of wool

b) Wool becomes loose, limp and straight

c) Enzootic ataxia

d) All of the above

25 Sway back disease is caused by

a) Nutritional deficiency of copper

b) Copper toxicity

c) Molybdenum deficiency

d) None of the above

26 Congenital swayback in lambs shows

a) Inability to stand b) Inability to suckle

c) Incoordinated movement d) All of the above

27 Enzootic ataxia is usually seen in age group of
a) 4-6 months b) 1-2 months
c) 3-4 months d) Adults

28 Clinical manifestation of enzootic ataxia includes
a) Excessive flexion of joints b) Knuckling of fetlock
c) Wobbling of hind legs d) All of the above

29 Enzootic ataxia has been seen in
a) Unweaned lambs b) Young goat kids
c) Pigs d) All of the above

30 Parenteral treatment of copper deficiency includes
a) Copper glycinate b) Copper sulphate
c) Molybdenate salt d) Sodium sulphate

31 Iodine deficiency is caused by
a) High intake of Ca
b) Diets consisting of Brassica sp.
c) Continuous intake of low level of cyanogenic glycoside
d) All of the above

32 Iodine is necessary as its deficiency may lead to
a) Decreased thyroxin production
b) Enlargement of thyroid gland
c) Hair abnormality
d) All of the above

33 Goitrogenic substances seen in pastures feed of animal
a) Linseed b) Kale
c) Rapeseed meal d) All of the above

34 Inherited form of goiter occursin cattle, due to
a) Goitrogenic feed of pregnant lamb
b) Increased ability of indotyrosine deiodinase enzyme
c) Both of the above
d) None of the above

35 Clinical signs of iodine deficiency are
a) Prolonged gestation in mare, cows and ewes
b) Partial or complete alopecia in different species

c) Reproductive abnormality

d) All of the above

36 Recommended dietary intake of iodine

a) 0.8 to 10 mg/kg of feed for lactating and pregnant cows

b) 0.1 to 0.3 mg/kg of feed for pregnant cows

c) Both of the above

d) 2-3 mg/kg of feed

37 Iron deficiency is mostly seen in young animals as

a) Milk is a poor sources of Fe

b) Deposits of in newborn is insufficient

c) Both of the above

d) None of the above

38 The most susceptible animal for Fe deficiency is

a) Horses b) Cattle

c) Sheep d) Pigs

39 Piglet anaemia is mostly seen in age group of

a) 5-6 week old b) 1-2 weeks old

c) 3-6 weeks old d) Above 8 weeks old

40 Preventive measure for piglet anaemia includes

a) Fe-Dextran injection in 24 hour old piglet

b) Painting the dams teat with Fe solution

c) Oral supplementation of dam before farrowing

d) All of the above

41 The cause of Fe deficiency

a) Ectoparasite infestation b) Strongylid infection

c) $CaCO_3$or Mn in diet d) All of the above

42 Clinical signs of Fe deficiency apart from anaemia

a) Mild diarrhoea b) Lethargy

c) Oedema of teat and fore quarters d) All of the above

43 Predisposing factors for NaCl deficiency

a) Hot weather b) Increased physical work

c) Grazing pasture in sandy soil d) All of the above

44 Manifestation of feeding Na deficient diet

a) Pica b) Rough hair coat

c) Drinking urine d) All of the above

45 Parakeratosis in pigs is due to mineral deficiency of

a) Copper b) Calcium

c) Zinc d) Magnesium

46 Clinical signs associated with zinc deficiency

a) Papules b) Erythema of skin & alopecia

c) Wool-eating in sheep d) All of the above

47 Differential diagnosis of Zn-responsive dermatitis

a) Sarcoptic mange b) Exudative dermatitis

c) Both (a) and (b) d) None of the above

48 An excess of which minerals increases Mn requirement

a) Ca b) Mg

c) P d) Both (a) and (b)

49 Clinical signs associated with Manganese deficiency

a) Infertility

b) Dry hair coat and loss of hair colour

c) Congenital chondrodystrophy

d) All of the above

50 Manganese interfers with the utilisation of

a) Cobalt b) Zinc

c) Molybdenum d) Both (a) and (b)

51 Mineral protecting the tissues from the oxidative damage is

a) Calcium b) Phosphorous

c) Selenium d) Potassium

52 Clinical disorders associated with selenium deficiency

a) Nutritional muscular distrophy b) Reproductive failure

c) Mulberry heart disease d) All of the above

53 Type of degeneration seen in "White Muscle Disease" due to selenium deficiency

a) Hydropic degeneration b) Zenker's degeneration

c) Wallerian degeneration d) Albuminous degeneration

54 Mulberry heart disease or yellow fat disease is commonly seen in

a) Cattle b) Pig
c) Horse d) Dogs

55 Calcium deficiency can be aggravated by high intake of

a) Copper b) Phosphorous
c) Zinc d) None of the above

56 Clinical symptoms associated with calcium deficiency

a) Poor development of gums and scisors
b) Tendency of bones to fracture
c) Difficulty in parturition
d) All of the above

57 Calcium deficiency results in

a) Rickets in growing animals b) Osteomalacia in adults
c) Degenerative arthropathy d) All of the above

58 Peri parturient haemoglobinuria is predisposed by deficiency of

a) Calcium b) Zinc
c) Magnesium d) Phosphorous

59 Pica, intake of unusual things by animals,is seen due to deficiency of

a) Phosphorous b) Calcium
c) Manganese d) Sulphur

60 The most susceptible animal to phosphorous deficiency

a) Horses b) Sheep
c) Cattle d) Goat

61 Clinical signs associated with phosphorous deficiency

a) Fracture of bones b) Impaired reproduction
c) Allotriophagia d) All of the above

62 Hypokalemia in cattle can occur secondarily to

a) GIT obstruction
b) Diarrhoea
c) Right side displacement or torsion of abomasum
d) All of the above

63 Hypokalemia is seen during administration of which of the following drugs, used for treatment of ketosis

a) Monensin
b) Isoflupridone
c) Niacin and Nicotinic acid
d) All of the above

64 Clinical signs associated with Vitamin-A deficiency

a) Microphthalmia in pig
b) Encephalopathy in calves
c) Thickening and hypersensitization of skin
d) All of the above

65 Organ system that is affected by hypovitaminosis-A

a) Reproductive System
b) Respiratory System
c) Gastrointestinal System
d) All of the above

66 Major causes of Vitamin-D deficiency

a) Inadequate UV radiation
b) Grazing on lush pasture
c) Vitamin-D deficient diet
d) All of the above

67 Vitamin-D is a necessary vitamin as it helps in

a) Eseprithaliazation
b) Absorption of Ca and P
c) Maintaining cell integrity
d) Immune response

68 Animal capable of synthesizing Vit-K in the intestine

a) Carnivorous
b) Ruminants only
c) Herbivorous
d) Avian

69 Vit-K plays an important role in

a) Erythropoiesis
b) Blood coagulation
c) Immune response
d) All of the above

70 Vitamin K is drug of choice in

a) Warfarin poisoning
b) Epistaxis
c) Haemorrhagic enteritis
d) All of the above

71 The most effective form of vitamin-E is

a) α-tocopherol
b) β-tocopherol
c) δ-tocopherol
d) All of the above

72 Clinical signs associated with Vit-E deficiency

a) Sterility b) Muscular degeneration

c) Mulberry heart in pig d) All of the above

73 Vit-E deficiency has clinical signs similar to that of

a) Sodium deficiency b) Magnesium Deficiency

c) Selenium Deficiency d) Vitamin A Deficiency

74 Vitamin -K helps in blood coagulation directly by

a) Formation of prothrombin b) Activation of fibrinogen

c) Formation of bile salt d) Both (a) and (b)

Answer Key

1	d	**2**	d	**3**	a	**4**	d	**5**	d	**6**	d	**7**	c	**8**	d	**9**	d	**10**	a
11	b	**12**	b	**13**	d	**14**	c	**15**	d	**16**	c	**17**	c	**18**	a	**19**	d	**20**	d
21	a	**22**	c	**23**	c	**24**	d	**25**	a	**26**	d	**27**	b	**28**	d	**29**	d	**30**	a
31	d	**32**	d	**33**	d	**34**	b	**35**	d	**36**	c	**37**	c	**38**	d	**39**	c	**40**	d
41	d	**42**	d	**43**	d	**44**	d	**45**	b	**46**	d	**47**	c	**48**	d	**49**	d	**50**	d
51	c	**52**	d	**53**	c	**54**	b	**55**	b	**56**	d	**57**	d	**58**	d	**59**	a	**60**	c
61	d	**62**	d	**63**	d	**64**	d	**65**	d	**66**	d	**67**	b	**68**	c	**69**	b	**70**	d
71	a	**72**	d	**73**	c	**74**	d												

18

Diseases of Neonates

1 Delayed post natal diseases occurs within _______ days after birth

a) 10 days b) 2-7 days

c) 2 days d) 15-30 days

2 White muscle disease and enterotoxemia comes under

a) Postnatal diseases b) Delayed postnatal diseases

c) Late post natal diseases d) Pre-natal diseases

3 Neonatal mortality in cow ranges from

a) Less than 3% b) 3-30%

c) More than 30% d) None of the above

4 Mortality of newborn is high due to

a) Hypothermia b) Poor mothering

c) No colostrum feeding d) All of the above

5 Congenital defect in newborn is seen due to

a) Viral disease b) Poisonous plants

c) Nutritional deficiency d) All of the above

6 Viruse scausing congenital defect are

a) Blue tongue virus b) Bovine viral disease

c) Rinderpest d) Both (a) and (b)

7 Mortality pattern of a herd depends upon

a) Type of housing b) Presence of attendant

c) Density of calves d) All the above

8 Enzootic ataxia in lambs occurs due to deficiency of

a) Iron b) Copper

c) Molybdenum d) Cobalt

9 Perinatal disease is classified into

a) Foetal disease
b) Parturient disease
c) Post natal disease
d) Delayed and postnatal disease

10 In case of piglets, the most common cause of mortality is

a) Infectious agents
b) Perinatal
c) Non infectious causes
d) All of the above

11 Lamb mortality generally occurs within

a) In the womb
b) During first month after birth
c) Non infectious diseases
d) All of the above

12 Eye defects and hare lips are seen due to deficiency of

a) Vit-A
b) Vit-B1
c) Vit-D
d) Vit-E

13 Limb deformities in calf is seen due to deficiency of

a) Selenium
b) Manganese
c) Copper
d) Molybdenum

Answer Key

1 b **2** c **3** b **4** d **5** d **6** d **7** d **8** b **9** c **10** c
11 d **12** a **13** b

19

Common Poisoning

1 Increased concentration of delta aminolevulinic acid is an indicator of toxicity due to

a) Lead b) Nitrate

c) Arsenic d) Cadmium

2 The drug of choice in case of rodenticide poisoning is

a) Atropine Sulphate b) Vit-K

c) Dexamethasone d) Doxapram

3 Diethyl phosphothionate (DETP) estimation in urine helps in detecting

a) Organochlorine b) Carbamate

c) Organophosphate d) DDT

4 Alkaline Phosphatase and glutamyl transferase are early indicators of toxicity involving

a) Liver b) Kidney

c) heart d) spleen

5 Nitrate poisoning is most common in

a) Cattle b) Sheep/Goat

c) Dog d) Both (a) and (b)

6 Chocolate brown colour mucus membrane is seen in toxicity due to

a) Nitrate/Nitrite b) Lead

c) Arsenic d) Mercury

7 Minimum lethal dose of nitrite in cattle is

a) 10-20 mg/kg body wt b) 40-50 mg/kg body wt

c) 20-30 mg/kg body wt d) 90-110 mg/kg body wt

8 Modified Diphenylamine test is carried out in poisonings due to for

a) Nitrate b) Lead

c) Sulphor d) Suipoisoning

9 Which of the following chemical in plants upon its ingestion leads to outbreak of HCN poisoning in animals

a) Glycosides b) Alkaloids

c) Tannins d) All of the above

10 Lead poisoning can be ameliarated by ingestions of

a) Sugarcane b) Linseed cake

c) Acacia, Sorghum, Sudangrass d) All of the above

11 Minimum lethal dose of cyanide in plants to induce cyanide poisoning in cattle, sheep, goat (mg/kg body wt.)

a) 2 b) 3

c) 5 d) 4

12 Chlorinated Napthalene, coaltar pitch, paraffin are

a) Hepatotoxic b) Cardiotoxic

c) Nephro toxic d) Neuro toxic

13 Mercury, lead, cadmium and ethylene glycol causes lesions in

a) Kidney b) Liver

c) Heart d) Respiratory System

14 Poisoning of H_2S, Ammonia oxides, Carbon etc. causes lesions in

a) Liver b) Heart

c) Kidney d) Respiratory System

15 Picrate paper test is used for diagnosis of

a) HCN poisoning b) Nitrate poisoning

c) Arsenic poisoning d) Mercury poisoning

16 Any substance that has potential to produce health hazard by its inherent chemical properties is called

a) Drug b) Toxicant

c) Poison d) All of the above

17 Hair coat depigmentation and secondary cuprosis is seen in

a) Copper toxicity b) Organo phosphate poisoning

c) Molybdenum toxicity d) Selenium toxicity

18 Laryngeal paralysis in horse is seen in poisoning with

a) Copper poisoning b) Cadmium poisoning

c) Molybdenum poisoning d) Agrochemicals

19 Universal antidote contains

a) 2 parts activated charcoal b) 1 part tannic acid

c) 1 part magnesium oxide d) All of the above

20 Antidote for mercury and arsenic poisoning

a) Calcium disodium EDTA b) BAL is British Antilewistic

c) Methylene Blue d) Sodium thiosulphate

Answer Key

1	a	**2**	b	**3**	c	**4**	b	**5**	d	**6**	a	**7**	d	**8**	a	**9**	a	**10**	d
11	a	**12**	a	**13**	a	**14**	d	**15**	a	**16**	b	**17**	c	**18**	a	**19**	c	**20**	b

20

Emergency Medicine and Critical Care

1 In emergency medicine, first aid measures do not include examination of

a) Airway b) Breathing

c) Circulation d) Blood Pressure

2 Which of the followings does not come under life threatening emergency

a) Severe haemorrhage b) Snake Bites

c) Poisoning d) Fractures

3 Which of the followings does not come under minor emergency

a) Dystokia b) Abscess

c) Insect sting d) Haematuria

4 Tachycardia occurs when heart rate exceeds _________ in dogs

a) 120-140 min b) 140-160 min

c) 150-170 min d) > 160-180 min

5 Normal Capillary refill time is

a) 0.5 sec b) 1-1.5 sec

c) 1 sec d) 2-3 sec

6 Capillary refill time of 3 seconds denotes

a) Serious vasoconstriction and poor perfusion

b) Dehydration

c) Shock

d) Cardiac Disease

7 Normal blood pressure (Systole: Diastole) in cattle is

a) 50: 80 b) 40:90

c) 30:70 d) 40:70

8 Vasodilator used in cardiogenic shock

a) Doxapram b) Nikethamide

c) Atropine d) Dopamine

9 Which is of the following is and menstured in showing brady cardia?

a) Atropine Sulphate b) Glycopyrolate
c) Xylazine d) Both (a) and (b)

10 Atropine sulphate is given in dog at dose rate of

a) 0.02 mg/kg b) 0.04 mg/kg
c) 0.04 mg/kg d) 0.01 mg/kg

11 Plasma and dextran are given in cardiac emergency at the dose rate of (ml/kg)

a) 40 b) 50
c) 20-30 d) 10-20

12 Congested mucous membrane is seen in which type of shock

a) Traumatic b) Hypovolemic
c) Septic d) Cardiogenic

13 Device/Instruments used to measure oxygenation and ventillation

a) Pulse oximeter b) Blood Gas analyser
c) Caprometry d) All of the above

14 Supplemental oxygen given in case of emergency at the dose rate of

a) 50-100 ml/kg/min b) 100 -200 ml/kg/min
c) 25-50 ml/kg/min d) 200 ml/kg/min

15 In case of burn the serum albumin and protein is to be kept between respectively

a) >2g/dl & 4-6.5 g/dl b) 5g/dl & 5g/dl
c) 5g/dl & 10g/dl d) 4-6.5 g/dl & 2g/dl

16 Escharectomy is performed in case of

a) Shock b) Severe haemorrhage
c) Chronic abcess d) Burn

17 Burn tissue is known as

a) Eschar b) Keloid
c) Sarcoid d) Gangrene

18 The best enema, easily available, is

a) Charcoal b) Luke warm water
c) Sodium bicarbonate d) Atropine sulphate

19 Cathartics are useful in

a) Elimination of Gas
b) Fecal Softner
c) Elimination of froth
d) Climination of toxins

20 Mineral oils as pugatives are to be administered in dogs in case of poisoning at the dote of (ml/kg) at the dose rate of (ml/kg)

a) 5-15
b) 20
c) 5
d) 25-30

Answer Key

1	d	**2**	d	**3**	a	**4**	d	**5**	b	**6**	a	**7**	b	**8**	d	**9**	d	**10**	b
11	c	**12**	c	**13**	d	**14**	a	**15**	a	**16**	d	**17**	a	**18**	b	**19**	a	**20**	a

21

Alternative Medicine in Animal Diseases Management

1 Many of active ingredients in chemically manmade drugs are derived from plant components

a) Pyrethroids b) Organophosphorous

c) Carbamate d) Organochlorine

2 What % of agricultural GDP is contributed by the livestock sector

a) 20 b) 32

c) 40 d) 25

3 First known Veterinary Doctor in the world around 1800 BC

a) Salihotra b) Nakula

c) Charak d) Palikapaya

4 Phenol acts as

a) Antiseptic b) Antiinflammatory

c) Antioxidant d) All of the above

5 Tannins acts as

a) Resistance to infection b) Astrigent

c) Antidiarroheal d) All of the above

6 Which is of the following compounds contains drugs like a tropine and vincrystine?

a) Phenol b) Alkaloids

c) Glycosides d) Flavoloids

7 Which is used for pigmentation of medicinal herbs

a) Ethylene oxide b) Formaldehyde

c) X-ray d) UV light

8 Overuse of Aloe vera juice can cause loss of

a) K^+ b) Na^+

c) Ca^{2+} d) Cl^-

9 Which of the followings has actions as anticoagulant and aspirin

a) Ginger b) Garlic

c) Turmeric d) Cardmon

10 Ethnoveterinary Medicine means

a) Use of traditional knowledge as a system

b) Folk beliefs

c) Skills, techniques and practices of traditional time

d) All of the above

11 What is fed to animals for getting more milk?

a) Gurmethi b) Gundijrans

c) Rice gruel d) All of the above

12 Poly herbal preparations used in GIT disorders

a) Neblon, Rumentaton b) HB strong

c) Rumbion, Appeved d) All of the above

13 Accacia catechu is obtained from which part of the plant

a) Root b) Leaves

c) Stem bark d) All of the above

14 *Allium sativum* bulb and tuber produces compound which act as

a) Carminative b) Diuretic

c) Astringent d) Both (a) and (b)

15 *Aloe vera* contains

a) Anthraquinoren b) Diuretic

c) Astringent d) Both (a) and (b)

16 Bignonia catalpa (Indian bean tree) bark and fruits act as

a) Sedative b) Stomachics

c) Antipyretics d) Antispasmodic

17 *Alium cepa* (Onion) bulb is used in

a) Carminative b) Purgation

c) Prolapse of uterus d) Astringent

18 Eucalyptus is used as

a) Antiseptic b) Expectorant

c) Carminative d) All of the above

19 Ficus bengalensis (Banyan tree) bark, leaves and roots acts as

a) Astringent b) Carminative

c) Abortifacient d) Antiseptic

20 *Moringa oleifera* (Drumstick) acts as

a) Abortifacient b) Antidote of Ach

c) Expectorant d) Carminative

21 Tulsi leaves act as

a) Antidiabetic b) Antibacterial

c) Expectorant d) All of the above

Answer Key

1 a **2** c **3** a **4** d **5** d **6** b **7** a **8** a **9** b **10** d

11 d **12** d **13** c **14** d **15** d **16** a **17** c **18** d **19** a **20** a

21 d

22

Bacterial Diseases

1 Which of the following diseases is also known as Equine Distemper?
   a) Eastern Equine Encephalomyelitis
   b) Western Equine Encephalomyelitis
   c) Strangles
   d) Glanders
2 The causative organism of Equine Distemper is
   a) *Streptococcus equi* subsp. *equi*
   b) *Streptococcus equi* var *zooepidemicus*
   c) *Pseudomonas mallei*
   d) *Streptococcus pseudointermedius*
3 Which of the following is the major source of infection in Strangles?
   a) Saliva b) Nasal discharge
   c) Discharge from the abscess d) Both (b) and (c)
4 Acute form of Strangles is characterized by each of the following except
   a) Abscessation of retropharyngeal lymph node
   b) Abscessation of submandibular lymph node
   c) Abscessation of prescapular lymphnode
   d) Mucopurulent nasal discharge
5 The common complications of strangles in horse is
   a) Bastard strangles / Metastatic infection
   b) Suppurative meningitis
   c) Suppurative necrotic bronchopneumonia
   d) All of the above
6 Which of the following occurs as a sequel to strangles in horse?
   a) Synchronous diaphragmatic flutter
   b) Purpura hemorrhagica

c) Disseminated intravascular coagulopathy
d) None of the above

7 The treatment of choice for *S. equi* infection (strangles) in horse is
a) Procaine penicillin G-22,000 IU/kg, q12 hr
b) Procaine penicillin G-44,000 IU/kg, q12 hr
c) Sodium or Potassium penicillin G-22,000 IU/kg, q6 hr
d) None of the above

8 Which of the following microbial protein is responsible for the tissue adhesion, invasion of pharyngeal tonsils as well as antiphagocytic activity of *S. equi* leading to initiation of clinical Strangles?
a) Beta-hemolysin b) M protein
c) Lethal protein d) All of the above

9 Caseous lymphadenitis in sheep and goat is caused by
a) *Mycobacterium paratuberculosis*
b) *Pseudomonas aeruginosa*
c) *Corynebacterium pseudotuberculosis*
d) *Corynebacterium pyogenes*

10 Common species affected with caseous lymphadenitis is
a) Sheep and goat b) Cattle and buffalo
c) Horse and mule d) Pig

11 During necropsy, the lamellated appearance of pus-filled abscess inside the superficial lymph nodes in sheep is the characteristic finding of
a) Tuberculosis b) Caseous lymphadenitis
c) Ulcerative lymphangitis d) Both (b) and (c)

12 Ulcerative lymphangitis in cattle and horse is caused by
a) *Corynebacterium pseudotuberculosis* biotype 1
b) *Corynebacterium pseudotuberculosis* biotype 2
c) Both (a) and (b)
d) *Streptococcus bovis*

13 In a horse affected with ulcerative lymphangitis, development of subcutaneous nodules and ulcers are usually restricted to which part of the body?
a) Neck b) Sub-mandibular region
c) Oral cavity d) Lower limb

14 The possible source of infection for anthrax in farm animals is

a) Infected soil and fodder grown on infected soil

b) Infected excreta, blood and other body discharge

c) Contaminated bone meals and hide

d) All of the above

15 Which of the following species are resistant to anthrax?

a) Algerian sheep b) Dwarf pig

c) Dog and Cat d) All of the above

16 Viability of anthrax bacilli increases in

a) Alkaline soil

b) Warm climate (temperature above 15°C)

c) Higher content of organic matter in soil

d) All of the above

17 The most common mode of transmission of anthrax in animals is

a) Inhalation b) Ingestion

c) Percutaneous d) Vector borne

18 *Bacillus anthracis* is resistant to phagocytosis due to the presence of

a) Poly-D-glutamic acid capsule b) Edema factor

c) Lethal toxin d) Protective antigen

19 In which species, anthrax always occurs as an acute form?

a) Cattle b) Pig

c) Horse d) Sheep

20 Which of the following stains is the best suitable for the detection of anthrax bacilli in peripheral blood smear?

a) Modified Zeihl-Neelson stain b) Polychrome methylene blue stain

c) PAS stain d) Levaditi's stain

21 Sawhorse posture of carcass is the characteristic finding of

a) Tetanus b) Brucellosis

c) Swine erysipelas d) Anthrax

22 Blackberry jam consistency of spleen is found in

a) Anthrax b) Tuberculosis

c) Paratuberculosis d) CBPP

23 Which of the following samples can be collected to confirm the diagnosis of anthrax in an unopened carcass?

a) Local edema fluid
b) Peripheral blood
c) Both of the above
d) None of the above

24 Ascolis test can be employed to detect the antigen of

a) *Clostridium tetany*
b) *Clostridium perfringens*
c) *Clostridium botulinum*
d) *Bacillus anthracis*

25 Which of the following statement regarding anthrax is false?

a) Veterinarians conducting postmortem examination of anthrax suspected carcass are susceptible to cutaneous anthrax
b) Shipping of the diagnostic sample through mail or courier system is strongly discouraged
c) Carcass should not be opened
d) None of the above

26 Hides, wool and mohair infected with anthrax spores should be sterilized by

a) Ethylene oxide
b) Gamma irradiation
c) 10% Formaldehyde
d) 5% Lysol

27 Preferred method for disposal of anthrax suspected carcass is

a) Incineration
b) Burial
c) Chemical treatment
d) None of the above

28 Which of the following statement is true regarding the immunization of animals with Stern avirulent spore vaccine of anthrax?

a) Immunity persists at least for 26 months in sheep and 1 year in cattle
b) No risk of development of anthrax after vaccination
c) Used in most countries now-a-days
d) All of the above

29 Animals vaccinated with anthrax vaccine should be withheld from slaughter for

a) 90 days
b) 60 days
c) 45 days
d) 7 days

30 During necropsy, subcutaneous swellings containing gelatinous material and enlargement of local lymph nodes at neck and pharynx region are the features of anthrax in which of the following species?

a) Sheep b) Horse

c) Pig d) Both (b) and (c)

31 The species mostly affected with listeriosis

a) Cattle b) Sheep

c) Goat d) Horse

32 Circling disease in sheep is caused by

a) *Listeria monocytogenes* b) *Leptospira interrogans*

c) *Clostridium botulinum* d) *Clostridium tetany*

33 In ruminants affected with listerial encephalitis, circling and head tilt is seen

a) On contralateral side

b) On ipsilateral side

c) Circling is ipsilateral while head tilt is

d) Circling is contralateral while head tilt is contra lateral ipsilateral

34 Circling movement, head tilt, unilateral facial hypolgesia and facial paralysis in sheep are the features of

a) Ovine ketosis b) Enterotoxaemia

c) Silagesickness d) Botulism

35 Listerial abortion is rarely seen in

a) Goat b) Cattle

c) Sheep d) Pig

36 In small ruminants, abortion due to listeriosis commonly occurs during

a) First 3 months of pregnancy

b) After 12th week of pregnancy

c) At any time during pregnancy

d) Abortion does not occur in small ruminants

37 In ovines, listerial encephalitis and abortion commonly occurs in

a) Outbreak form b) Sporadic form

c) Pandemic form d) None of the above

38 Septicemic form of listeriosis is uncommon in
a) Lambs b) Calves
c) Adult cattle and sheep d) Pigs

39 Which of the followings is not seen in listeriosis in ruminants?
a) Spinal myelitis b) Ophthalmitis / Uveitis
c) Encephalitis and Meningitis d) None of the above

40 In listerial encephalitis, cerebrospinal fluid has
a) Increased protein concentration b) Increased leukocyte count
c) Both of the above d) None of the above

41 Which of the following diseases is associated with microabscessation of the CNS histological examination?
a) Rabies b) Listeriosis
c) Botulism d) Bovine Spongiform Encephalopathy

42 The dose of Penicillin for the treatment of listeriosis in ruminants is
a) 22000 IU/kg b) 44000 IU/kg
c) 66000 IU/kg d) 120000 IU/kg

43 Sudden death, diamond shaped skin lesions, arthritis and endocarditis in swine is characteristic feature of
a) Classical swine fever b) African swine fever
c) Swine erysipelas d) Hog cholera

44 Swine erysipelas does not occur in which of the following form?
a) Hyperacute form b) Acute form
c) Sub-acute form d) Chronic form

45 Dark purple coloured diamond shaped skin lesion commonly occurs in which form of swine erysipelas.
a) Hyperacute b) Acute
c) Sub-acute d) Chronic

46 Non-suppurative proliferative arthritis and vegetative endocarditis are the characteristic of __________ form of swine erysipelas.
a) Hyperacute b) Acute
c) Sub-acute d) Chronic

47 In cattle affected with actinomycosis, swelling of the mandible or maxilla commences at the level of teeth.
a) 1st premolar b) 2nd premolar
c) 3rd premolar d) Central molar

48 Which of the followings is incorrect about lumpy jaw in cattle?

a) Rarefying osteomyelitis of mandible and maxilla

b) Bony swellings are painful initially and painless in later stages

c) Pus is honey like and contains yellow-white granules

d) Lymph nodes are not affected

49 The soft tissue that is most commonly affected with actinomycosis in cattle is

a) Tongue b) Liver

c) Esophageal groove d) Small intestine

50 The presence of club colonies containing thread like bacteria in the smear made from crushed granules of the pus is characteristic feature of

a) Actinomycosis b) Tuberculosis

c) Glanders d) Ulcerative lymphangitis

51 Wooden tongue in cattle is caused by

a) *Actinobacillus seminis* b) *Actinobacillus lignieresii*

c) *Actinobacillus capsulatus* d) All of the above

52 Which of the followings is incorrect about actinobacillosis in cattle?

a) Causative organism is a normal inhabitant of oral cavity and rumen

b) Grazing with abrasive pasture is the major risk factor

c) Lymph nodes are not affected

d) Commonly involves the soft tissues

53 Which of the following organ is usually not affected in sheep with actinobacillosis?

a) Tongue b) Lower jaw

c) Nose d) Face

54 Which of the following is considered as a standard treatment for actinobacillosis in cattle?

a) Oxytetracycline b) Chloramphenicol

c) Potassium iodide d) Aminoglycosides

55 Which of the following is not a possible method of transmission of tuberculosis?

a) Inhalation and ingestion b) Intrauterine infection at coitus

c) Intramammary infection d) None of the above

56 Non-progressive form of tuberculosis is seen in which species?

a) Sheep b) Goat

c) Horse d) Pig

57 Tuberculosis is progressive in which species?

a) Cattle b) Horse

c) Sheep and goat d) All of the above

58 Noisy breathing in animals affected with tuberculosis is due to

a) Accumulation of fluid in trachea

b) Constriction of bronchi

c) Enlargement of retropharyngeal lymphnode causing pharyngeal obstruction

d) Pleurisy

59 Pearl disease is the synonym of __________.

a) Brucellosis b) Tuberculosis

c) Paratuberculosis d) Dermatophytosis

60 Which of the following diseases is associated with amber colour fluid accumulation at the top of the milk upon allowed to stand is found in?

a) Tuberculous mastitis b) Leptospiral mastitis

c) Mycoplasmal mastitis d) Staphylococcal mastitis

61 Painful osteomyelitis of cervical vertebrae causing stiffness of the neck in horse is seen in which of the following bacterial diseases?

a) Actinomycosis b) Tetanus

c) Botulism d) Tuberculosis

62 The commonest form of tuberculosis in small ruminants is

a) Tuberculous mastitis b) Bronchopneumonia

c) Interstitial pneumonia d) Tuberculous metritis

63 Which of the followings is not a test for detection of tuberculosis in animals?

a) Stormont test b) Short thermal test

c) SID test d) Sabin fieldman dye test

64 The type of hypersensitivity reaction, shown by the affected animals in SID test for the detection of tuberculosis

a) Type I b) Type II

c) Type III d) Type IV

65 The dose of tuberculin administered to the animal in SID test is

a) 0.1 ml b) 0.2 ml

c) 0.5 ml d) 1 ml

66 In SID test, the reaction should be read between _____ hours after injection.

a) 24-48 b) 48-72

c) 72-96 d) 96-120

67 The maximum permissible rate of NVL reactors in SID test is

a) 5% b) 10%

c) 15% d) 20%

68 Which of the followings is the disadvantage of SID test?

a) Lack of specificity

b) No Visible-lesion reactors (NVLs)

c) Failure to detect the disease in old and recently calved cows

d) All of the above

69 The route of administration of tuberculin injection in Stormont test is

a) Intradermal b) Subcutaneous

c) Intramuscular d) Intravenous

70 An animal is said to be positive in Stormont test if the increase in the skin thickness is more than

a) 1 mm b) 2 mm

c) 3 mm d) 5 mm

71 The animals with visible lesions of tuberculosis but not reacting to intradermal tuberculin test are known as

a) No Visible-lesion reactors b) Floaters

c) Anergic animals d) All of the above

72 Nodules or tubercles in the intestinal wall, spleen and mesenteric lymph nodes is a characteristic necropsy finding in which species?

a) Goat b) Horse

c) Pig d) Buffalo

73 Which species is most commonly affected with Johne's disease?

a) Cattle b) Buffalo

c) Sheep d) Goat

74 The most common route of exposure of a calf to causative organism of paratuberculosis is

a) Ingestion of urine contaminated feed and water

b) Direct contact with nasal and oral secretions of infected animals

c) Nursing from an infected dam

d) Intrauterine exposure

75 The primary site of multiplication of *Mycobacterium paratuberculosis* in cattle is

a) Terminal part of small intestine b) Large intestine

c) Both a and b d) Only at cecum

76 The clinical signs of paratuberculosis are most commonly seen in cattle of age group

a) 6 month-1year b) 1-2 year

c) 2-6 year d) 6-10 year

77 Cattle passing thick pea soup like faeces without any offensive order is seen in

a) Johne's disease b) Fasciolosis

c) Salmonellosis d) Coccidiosis

78 In which stage of paratuberculosis, diarrhoea is characterized by a fluid 'water hose' or pipe stream passage of faeces?

a) Silent infection b) Subclinical stage

c) Clinical stage d) Advanced clinical stage

79 Johnin test is applied for the diagnosis of which disease?

a) Actinomycosis b) Actinobacillosis

c) Paratuberculosis d) Tuberculosis

80 In which of the following diseases, thickened intestinal wall with corrugated mucosa is a characteristic necropsy finding?

a) Haemonchosis b) Paratuberculosis

c) Coccidiosis d) Clostridial infection

81 In animals affected with JD, the part of intestine which appears corrugated is

a) Terminal part of small intestine b) Caecum

c) First part of colon d) All of the above

82 Strawberry foot rot in sheep is caused by

a) *Staphylococcus aureus* b) *Dermatophillus congolensis*

c) *Staphylococcus hyicus* d) *Streptococcus pyogenes*

83 Glanders in horse is caused by

a) *Streptococcus equi* b) *Actinobacillus equi*

c) *Pseudomonas mallei* d) *Pseudomonas pseudomallei*

84 Which form of glanders, the horses mostly develop

a) Per-acute b) Acute

c) Sub-acute d) Chronic

85 Mules and donkeys commonly develop which form of glanders

a) Per-acute b) Acute

c) Sub-acute d) Chronic

86 The organism of which of the following diseases is used as an agent of bioterrorism?

a) Strangles b) Glanders

c) Tuberculosis d) Brucellosis

87 The main cause of death in horse affected with glanders is

a) Asphyxia b) Coma

c) Anoxic anoxia d) Histotoxic anoxia

88 Which of the following form of glanders is seen in horse?

a) Pulmonary form b) Nasal form

c) Skin form d) All of the above

89 Which of the following statements is incorrect about glanders?

a) In nasal form of the disease, the lesions appear in nasal septum and lower part of turbinate

b) Ulcers in the nasal mucosa are replaced by stellate scars

c) Farcy pipes are characteristic

d) None of the above

90 A horse is presented with purulent blood-stained nasal discharge with laboured breathing, discharge of dark honey coloured pus from the skin nodules and thickened lymph vessels radiating from the skin lesions. Which of the following disease is most likely the horse affected with?

a) Strangles b) Glanders

c) Ulcerative lymphangitis d) Epizootic lymphangitis

91 Mallein test is done for the diagnosis of

a) Melioidosis b) Caseous lymphadenitis

c) Glanders d) Ulcerative lymphangitis

92 The dose and route of administration of mallein in mallein test are

a) 0.1 ml, sub-cutaneous b) 0.1 ml, intradermal

c) 1 ml, sub-cutaneous d) 1 ml, intradermal

93 The site of intradermal injection in mallein test is

a) Neck b) Lower eye lid

c) Base of tail d) None of the above

94 Which of the following test cannot be used for diagnosis glanders?

a) Mallein test b) CFT

c) Strauss reaction d) None of the above

95 The laboratory animal used to elicit the strauss reaction for diagnosis of glanders in horse is

a) Rat b) Mice

c) Guinea pig d) Hamster

96 Which of the followings should be considered as differential diagnosis for glanders?

a) Epizootic lymphangitis b) Ulcerative lymphangitis

c) Sporotrichosis d) All of the above

97 The source of infection in the spread of leptospirosis is

a) Infected urine b) Uterine discharge

c) Aborted fetus d) All of the above

98 Abortion storm in cattle herd may occur in which form of leptospirosis?

a) Acute b) Sub-acute

c) Chronic d) Per-acute

99 Abortion in sheep is a manifestation of which form of leptospirosis?

a) Acute b) Sub-acute

c) Chronic d) Per-acute

100 Which type of nephritis is the characteristic of leptospirosis?

a) Glomerulonephritis b) Interstitial nephritis

c) Pyelonephritis d) All of the above

101 Encephalitis due to localization of leptospirae in nervous tissue commonly occurs in

a) Horse b) Pig

c) Sheep and goat d) Dog

102 Which species is commonly affected with recurrent uveitis due to leptospirosis?

a) Buffalo b) Horse

c) Pig d) Dog

103 Hemolytic anemia with hemoglobinuria, jaundice and fever in cattle are the clinical findings of

a) Leptospirosis b) Babesiosis

c) Bacillary hemoglobinuria d) All of the above

104 Appearance of blood stained or yellow-orange colored milk from all the four quarters without any physical change in the udder of cattle is seen in

a) *Clostridium hemolyticum* infection

b) Streptococcal mastitis

c) Gangrenous mastitis

d) Leptospiral mastitis

105 Abortion in cattle due to leptospirosis usually occurs in ______ trimester of pregnancy.

a) 1st b) 2nd

c) 3rd d) At any time of pregnancy

106 The most commonly used serological test for the diagnosis of leptospirosis is

a) AGID test b) CFT

c) FAT d) MAT

107 A MAT titer of ________ is considered positive for leptospiral infection.

a) ≥ 1:10 b) ≥ 1:20

c) ≥ 1:50 d) ≥ 1:100

108 Which type of antibodies against leptospira is detected in the serum by the microscopic agglutination test (MAT)?

a) IgM b) IgG

c) IgA d) Both a and b

109 Dark field microscopic examination of urine is used for the diagnosis of

a) Leptospirosis
b) Kidney worm infection
c) Babesiosis
d) Nocardiosis

110 The dose of dihydrostreptomycin adminstered for the elimination of leptospiruria in cattle is

a) 10 mg/kg
b) 12 mg/kg
c) 25 mg/kg
d) 50 mg/kg

111 Lyme disease in cattle is caused by

a) *Borrelia anserina*
b) *Borrelia burgdorferi*
c) *Borrelia recurrentis*
d) *Borrelia vincentii*

112 Marbling of lungs in cattle is the characteristic PM finding in

a) CCPP
b) CBPP
c) TB
d) All of the above

113 Contagious bovine pleuro pneumonia (CBPP) is caused by

a) *Mycoplasma mycoides*
b) *Mycoplasma bovis*
c) *Mycoplasma capricolium*
d) *Mycobacterium bovis*

114 Contagious caprine pleuro pneumonia (CCPP) is caused by

a) *Mycoplasma hypopneumoniae*
b) *Mycoplasma bovis*
c) *Mycoplasma capricolum*
d) *Mycobacterium bovis*

115 Infectious keratoconjunctivitis in sheep and goat is also known as

a) Pink eye
b) Contagious conjunctivo-keratitis
c) Contagious ophthalmia
d) All of the above

116 Pink eye in sheep is caused by

a) *Mycoplasma capri*
b) *Mycoplasma conjunctivae*
c) *Mycoplasma bovis*
d) *Mycoplasma capricolum*

117 In a sheep affected with contagious ophthalmia, corneal opacity is initially most pronounced at

a) Center of cornea
b) Ventral corneal-scleral junction
c) Dorsal corneal-scleral junction
d) Periphery of cornea

118 Septicemic pasteurellosis of cattle is associated with infection of

a) *Pasteurella multocida* biotype A

b) *Pasteurella multocida* biotype B

c) *Pasteurella hemolytica*

d) None of the above

119 Pneumonic pasteurellosis of cattle is associated with infection of

a) *Pasteurella multocida* biotype A

b) *Pasteurella multocida* biotype B

c) *Pasteurella hemolytica*

d) None of the above

120 Barbone disease is the synonym of

a) Hemorrhagic septicemia b) Pneumonic pasteurellosis

c) Septicemic pasteurellosis d) Both (a) and (c)

121 Which serotype of *P. multocida* causes most outbreaks of hemorrhagic septicemia in India?

a) B1 b) B2

c) D d) E2

122 What age group of cattle is more susceptible to hemorrhagic septicemia?

a) 2-6 month b) 6-9 month

c) 6 month 2 years d) 2-5 years

123 Outbreaks of hemorrhagic septicemia are most commonly seen in the season ___________.

a) Summer season b) Rainy season

c) Winter season d) Spring season

124 Hemorrhagic septicemia is characterized by

a) Sudden onset of fever

b) Severe dyspnoea

c) Painful swelling of dewlap and brisket

d) All of the above

125 Bang's disease is caused by

a) *Brucella abortus* b) *Brucella mellitensis*

c) *Brucella ovis* d) *Brucella suis*

126 Malta fever or Mediterranean fever is caused by

a) *Brucella abortus* b) *Brucella mellitensis*

c) *Brucella ovis* d) *Brucella suis*

127 Which of the following statements is incorrect about brucellosis in animals?

a) Sexually immature cattle are more susceptible than sexually mature cattle of either sex

b) Risk of disease transmission is high when semen from infected bull is used for artificial insemination

c) Ewes are more resistant than ram

d) A zoonotic disease

128 The substance produced by the fetus of animals infected with brucellosis and responsible for the growth of *Brucella abortus* is known as

a) Mycolic acid b) Erythritol

c) Alpha-hydroxylase d) Beta-hydroxylase

129 Abortion due to brucellosis principally occurs during

a) First 3 months of pregnancy b) Last 3 months of pregnancy

c) Mid pregnancy d) At any time during pregnancy

130 Orchitis and epididymitis in bull is characteristic feature of

a) Anthrax b) Black quarter

c) Brucellosis d) Hemorrhagic septicemia

131 Which among the following tests can be used for the screening of herds for brucellosis?

a) Milk ring test b) Rose Bengal plate test

c) Bruc ELISA d) All of the above

132 Necrotizing placentitis and disseminated inflammatory reactions in aborted fetus are the characteristic PM findings in

a) Trichomonosis b) Neosporosis

c) Brucellosis d) Leptospirosis

133 Strain 19 vaccine and strain RB51 vaccine are used for immunization of animals against

a) Anthrax b) Brucellosis

c) Trypanosomiasis d) Black quarter

134 Calfhood vaccination is associated with which of the following disease?

a) FMD b) Anthrax

c) Brucellosis d) Rabies

135 Pink eye in cattle is caused by

a) *Mycoplasma bovis* b) *Moraxella bovis*

c) *Histophilus somni* d) *Streptococcus bovis*

136 Tick pyemia of lambs is caused by

a) *Staphylococcus aureus*

b) *Staphylococcus intermedius*

c) *Staphylococcus pseudointermedius*

d) *Staphylococcus hyicus*

137 Exudative epidermitis or Greasy pig disease in swine is caused by

a) *Staphylococcus aureus*

b) *Staphylococcus intermedius*

c) *Staphylococcus pseudointermedius*

d) *Staphylococcus hyicus*

138 Periodic ophthalmia or moon blindness in horse is caused by

a) *Leptospira pomona*

b) *Leptospira hardzo*

c) *Leptospira icterohemorrhagica*

d) *Leptospira grippotyphosa*

139 Abortion storm in cattle is caused by

a) *Leptospira Pomona*

b) *Leptospira hardzo*

c) *Leptospira icterohemorrhagica*

d) *Leptospira grippotyphosa*

140 Which of the followings is a synonym of anthrax?

a) Spleenic fever b) Charbon

c) Malignant pustular dermatitis d) All of the above

141 The dose and route of administration of anthrax spore vaccine in domestic animals are

a) 1 ml, subcutaneous b) 3 ml, intramuscular

c) 5 ml, intravenous d) 10 ml, subcutaneous

142 The dose of anthrax spore vaccine in elephant is

a) 1 ml b) 3 ml

c) 5 ml d) 10 ml

143 Cold mastitis is caused by

a) *Staphylococcus* spp. b) *Streptococcus* spp.

c) *Leptospira* spp. d) *Mycoplasma* spp.

144 Weil's disease is also known as

a) Paratuberculosis b) Leptospirosis

c) Listeriosis d) Dirofilariasis

145 Leptospiral organism can be seen in tissue section by staining with

a) Bipolar stain

b) Diff Quick stain

c) Loeffler's methylene blue stain

d) Silver impregnation stain

146 The site of intradermal injection for the diagnosis of tuberculosis in pigs

a) Neck b) Shoulder

c) Ear d) Back

147 The organism of which of the following diseases can be visualized by bipolar staining?

a) Tuberculosis b) Paratuberculosis

c) Hemorrhagic septicemia d) Black quarter

148 Lung plague or lung sickness in cattle is the synonym of

a) Hemorrhagic septicemia b) CBPP

c) Tuberculosis d) Aspergillosis

149 Which of the followings is the synonym of black quarter?

a) Quarter ill b) Emphysematous gangrene

c) Symptomatic anthrax d) All of the above

150 Which of the followings is known as big head disease?

a) Gas gangrene b) Malignant edema

c) Both (a) and (b) d) Botulism

151 Black quarter is caused by

a) *Clostridium septicum* b) *Clostridium chauvoei*

c) *Clostridium botulinum* d) *Clostridium haemolyticum*

152 Braxy or Bradshot is caused by

a) *Clostridium septicum* b) *Clostridium chauvoei*

c) *Clostridium botulinum* d) *Clostridium haemolyticum*

153 Bacillary hemoglobinuria in cattle and sheep is caused by

a) *Clostridium septicum* b) *Clostridium chauvoei*

c) *Clostridium botulinum* d) *Clostridium haemolyticum*

154 Limber neck in domestic animals is caused by

a) *Clostridium septicum* b) *Clostridium chauvoei*

c) *Clostridium botulinum* d) *Clostridium haemolyticum*

155 Which of the followings is known as Saw horse disease?

a) Tetanus b) Botulism

c) Rickets d) Rabies

156 Lamb dysentery in young lambs is caused by

a) *Clostridium perfringens* type A

b) *Clostridium perfringens* type B

c) *Clostridium perfringens* type C

d) *Clostridium perfringens* type D

157 Struck in adult sheep is caused by

a) *Clostridium perfringens* type A

b) *Clostridium perfringens* type B

c) *Clostridium perfringens* type C

d) *Clostridium perfringens* type D

158 Pulpy kidney disease in sheep and goat is caused by

a) *Clostridium perfringens* type A

b) *Clostridium perfringens* type B

c) *Clostridium perfringens* type C

d) *Clostridium perfringens* type D

159 Hemorrhagic enterotoxaemia in piglets is caused by

a) *Clostridium perfringens* type A

b) *Clostridium perfringens* type B

c) *Clostridium perfringens* type C

d) *Clostridium perfringens* type D

160 Enterotoxaemia of foals is caused by

a) *Clostridium perfringens* type A

b) *Clostridium perfringens* type B

c) *Clostridium perfringens* type C

d) Both b and c

161 Calf enterotoxaemia is caused by

a) *Clostridium perfringens* type A

b) *Clostridium perfringens* type B

c) *Clostridium perfringens* type C

d) Both b and c

162 Bulbar paralysis or lame sickness is caused by.

a) *Clostridium botulinum* type C

b) *Clostridium botulinum* type D

c) *Clostridium novyi* type B

d) *Clostridium novyi* type D

163 Limberneck is caused by

a) *Clostridium botulinum* type C

b) *Clostridium botulinum* type D

c) *Clostridium novyi* type B

d) *Clostridium novyi* type D

164 Black leg in cattle is caused by

a) *Clostridium chauvoei*

b) *Clostridium botulinum* type C

c) *Clostridium novyi* type B

d) *Clostridium novyi* type D

165 Black disease is caused by

a) *Clostridium botulinum* type D

b) *Clostridium botulinum* type C

c) *Clostridium novyi* type B

d) *Clostridium novyi* type D

166 Tyzzer's disease is caused by

a) *Clostridium septicum* b) *Clostridium piliforme*

c) *Clostridium botulinum* d) *Clostridium haemolyticum*

167 Black disease is also known as

a) Black quarter b) Infectious keratitis
c) Infectious necrotic hepatitis d) Pulpy kidney disease

168 Black quarter is a _________ disease.

a) Water borne b) Vector borne
c) Air borne d) Soil borne

169 In enzootic area, primary vaccination with black quarter in cattle should be done at age of age in cattle.

a) 1 month b) 2 months
c) 6 months d) 12 months

170 A male kid is presented with clinical signs of bloat, muscle stiffness and locked jaw condition. There is a history of open method of castration. The disease with which the kid is most likely affected.

a) Cranial nerve deficit b) Facial nerve paralysis
c) Tetanus d) Listeriosis

171 The neurotoxin produced by *Clostridium tetani* is

a) Tetanolysin b) Tetanospasmin
c) Fibrinolysin d) All of the above

172 In tetanus affected animals, death occurs due to

a) Anoxia b) Coma
c) Syncope d) Asphyxia

173 Drum stick appearance spore is the characteristic feature of the organism of which disease.

a) Tetanus b) Botulism
c) Black quarter d) Enterotoxemia

174 Subcutaneous edema is not a feature of black quarter in ______ species.

a) Cattle b) Sheep
c) Both of the above d) None of the above

175 The predominant organism causing mastitis in farm animals is

a) *Streptococcus agalactiae* b) *Streptococcus dysgalactiae*
c) *Staphylococcus aureus* d) *E. coli*

176 Which of the following bacteria cause opportunistic mastitis?

a) *Staphylococcus warneri* b) *Staphylococcus simulans*
c) *Staphylococcus epidermidis* d) All of the above

177 The stage in the development of mastitis at which the pathogens move from the teat orifice into the teat canal is known as ______.

a) Infection b) Invasion

c) Inflammation d) Initiation

178 In a healthy lactating mammary gland, the somatic cell count (SCC) is

a) < 100 cells/ml b) < 1000 cells/ml

c) < 1,00,000 cells/ml d) < 10,00,000 cells/ml

179 Organism responsible for recurrent mastitis are

a) *Staphylococcus aureus* b) *Streptococcus dysgalactiae*

c) *Streptococcus agalactiae* d) Both a and b

180 Organism responsible for persistent mastitis are _________.

a) *Streptococcus agalactiae* b) *Streptococcus dysgalactiae*

c) *Mycobacterium bovis* d) Both a and c

181 The organism which is not commonly associated with contagious mastitis?

a) *Streptococcus agalactiae* b) *Streptococcus dysgalactiae*

c) *Mycobacterium bovis* d) *Staphylococcus aureus*

182 The most common mode of transmission of mastitis within a herd is ____.

a) Inhalation b) Milkers hands

c) Ingestion d) Through cutaneous injury

183 In tuberculous mastitis, the entry of organism into the mammary gland is mainly occurs through __________ route.

a) Intramammary b) Inhalation

c) Hematogenous d) Through cutaneous injury

184 The common mode of transmission of fungal mastitis is _________.

a) Intramammary infusion b) Inhalation

c) Hematogenous d) Through cutaneous injury

185 The common mode of transmission of mycoplasmal mastitis is _______.

a) Intramammary b) Inhalation

c) Hematogenous d) Through cutaneous injury

186 The iron binding protein present in milk which inhibits the growth of bacteria is ________ .

a) Hemoglobin b) Ferritin

c) Transferrin d) Lactoferrin

187 Gangrenous mastitis is caused by ___________ .

a) *Corynebacterium pyogenes* b) *Staphylococcus aureus*
c) *E. coli* d) *Streptococcus agalactiae*

188 Environmental mastitis is caused by __________ .

a) *Corynebacterium pyogenes* b) *Staphylococcus aureus*
c) *E. coli* d) *Streptococcus agalactiae*

189 Summer mastitis is caused by __________ .

a) *Corynebacterium pyogenes* b) *Staphylococcus aureus*
c) *E. coli* d) *Streptococcus agalactiae*

190 The type of mastitis in which the udder is enlarged, hard and painful is

a) Acute b) Chronic
c) Subclinical d) Subacute

191 The type of mastitis in which the udder is shrunken, hard but painless is

a) Acute b) Chronic
c) Subclinical d) Subacute

192 Bread-butter or shaggy appearance of affected quarter occurs in mastitis due to _________.

a) *Mycobacterium bovis* b) *Staphylococcus aureus*
c) *Pseudomonas aeruginosa* d) *Streptococcus agalactiae*

193 When milk is allowed to stand, there is deposition of amber colored fluid at the top. This indicates __________ mastitis.

a) Mycoplasmal b) Tuberculous
c) Leptospiral d) Coliform

194 When milk is allowed to stand, there is deposition of turbid whey colored fluid at the top. This indicates _________ mastitis.

a) Mycoplasmal b) Tuberculous
c) Leptospiral d) Coliform

195 Putrid odour of milk is the feature of mastitis due to __________ .

a) *Mycobacterium bovis* b) *Streptococcus agalactiae*
c) *Corynebacterium pyogenes* d) *Pseudomonas aeruginosa*

196 Bluish or greenish tinged milk is due to the infection of udder with______.

a) *Mycobacterium bovis* b) *Streptococcus agalactiae*
c) *Corynebacterium pyogenes* d) *Pseudomonas aeruginosa*

197 Abnormal milk comes at the end of milking in which of the following mastitis

a) Mycoplasmal mastitis b) Tuberculous mastitis
c) Leptospiral mastitis d) Coliform mastitis

198 Electrical conductivity of mastitis milk is increased due to increase in the concentration of _________ in milk.

a) Na^+ b) Cl^-
c) Ca++ d) Both (a) and (b)

199 Which of the following reagents is used in White side test for detection of mastitis?

a) Sodium carbonate b) Sodium bicarbonate
c) Sodium hydroxide d) Magnesium hydroxide

200 Hotis test is done to identify the presence of which organism in milk?

a) *Streptococcus agalactiae*
b) *Streptococcus dysgalactiae*
c) *Streptococcus zooepidemicus*
d) *Streptococcus pyogenes*

201 The most reliable cowside test for detecting subclinical mastitis is ______.

a) Hotis test b) CMT
c) NAGase test d) White side test

202 The pH indicator present in CMT reagent is___________.

a) Triethanolamine sulphonate b) Sodium lauryl sulphate (SLS)
c) Bromocresol purple d) Sodium hydroxide

203 In modified CMT, sodium lauryl sulphate (SLS) is used as __________.

a) pH indicator b) Detergent
c) Coloring agent d) None of the above

204 The best method for permanently drying off a quarter is infusion of______.

a) 5% Povidone iodine b) 1% Lugol's iodine
c) Dilute HCl d) 1% Copper sulphate

205 In dry cow therapy, the antimicrobial is administered during_____ to prevent mastitis.

a) Dry period
b) Lactation period
c) Immediately after the last milking of lactation
d) At the end of dry period

206 Lactating cow therapy is associated with mastitis due to __________.

a) *Staphylococcus aureus* b) *Streptococcus agalactiae*
c) *Corynebacterium pyogenes* d) *Pseudomonas aeruginosa*

207 Blitz therapy is performed in mastitis due to__________ .

a) *Staphylococcus aureus* b) *Streptococcus agalactiae*
c) *Corynebacterium pyogenes* d) *Pseudomonas aeruginosa*

208 Fowl typhoid is caused by__________ .

a) *Pasteurella multocida* b) *Salmonella pullorum*
c) *Salmonella gallinarum* d) *Salmonella enteritidis*

209 Fowl paratyphoid is caused by__________ .

a) *Pasteurella multocida* b) *Salmonella pullorum*
c) *Salmonella gallinarum* d) *Salmonella enteritidis*

210 Fowl cholera is caused by__________ .

a) *Pasteurella multocida* b) *Salmonella pullorum*
c) *Salmonella gallinarum* d) *Salmonella enteritidis*

211 Baby chick disease or bacillary white diarrhoea of chicks is caused by__________.

a) *Pasteurella multocida* b) *Salmonella pullorum*
c) *Salmonella gallinarum* d) *Salmonella enteritidis*

212 Chronic respiratory disease in chickens is caused by__________.

a) *Haemophilus gallinarum* b) *Mycoplasma gallisepticum*
c) *Mycoplasma synoviae* d) *Pasteurella multocida*

213 Infectious sinusitis in turkey is caused by__________.

a) *Haemophilus gallinarum* b) *Mycoplasma gallisepticum*
c) *Mycoplasma synoviae* d) *Pasteurella multocida*

214 Infectious synovitis is caused by__________.

a) *Haemophilus gallinarum* b) *Mycoplasma gallisepticum*
c) *Mycoplasma synoviae* d) *Pasteurella multocida*

215 Infectious coryza in poultry is caused by

a) *Haemophilus gallinarum* b) *Mycoplasma gallisepticum*
c) *Mycoplasma synoviae* d) *Pasteurella multocida*

216 Copper colored liver in chicken is the characteristic PM finding in __________.

a) Fowl cholera b) Fowl plague
c) Fowl paratyphoid d) Fowl typhoid

217 Whitish diarrhoea in chicks is the feature of which of the following diseases
  a) Fowl cholera b) Pullorum disease
  c) Fowl paratyphoid d) Fowl typhoid

218 Diarrhoea with blood-tinged faeces in affected birds is seen in
  a) Fowl cholera b) Pullorum disease
  c) Fowl paratyphoid d) Fowl typhoid

219 Fowl smelling discharges from the eyes and nostrils in chicken is seen in
  a) Infectious sinusitis b) Infectious synovitis
  c) Infectious coryza d) Infectious keratoconjunctivitis

220 Creamy or cheesy exudates in the synovial sac of hock joints, foot pad and on the skull is seen during necropsy of chicken affected with__________.
  a) Infectious sinusitis b) Infectious synovitis
  c) Infectious coryza d) Infectious kerato conjunctivitis

Answer Key

1 c	**2** a	**3** d	**4** c	**5** d	**6** b	**7** d	**8** b	**9** c	**10** a
11 b	**12** b	**13** d	**14** d	**15** d	**16** d	**17** b	**18** a	**19** c	**20** b
21 d	**22** a	**23** c	**24** d	**25** d	**26** b	**27** a	**28** d	**29** c	**30** d
31 b	**32** a	**33** b	**34** c	**35** d	**36** b	**37** a	**38** c	**39** d	**40** c
41 b	**42** b	**43** c	**44** c	**45** b	**46** d	**47** d	**48** b	**49** c	**50** a
51 b	**52** c	**53** a	**54** c	**55** d	**56** d	**57** d	**58** c	**59** b	**60** a
61 d	**62** b	**63** d	**64** d	**65** a	**66** b	**67** b	**68** d	**69** a	**70** d
71 c	**72** b	**73** a	**74** c	**75** c	**76** c	**77** a	**78** d	**79** c	**80** b
81 d	**82** b	**83** c	**84** d	**85** b	**86** b	**87** c	**88** d	**89** d	**90** b
91 c	**92** b	**93** b	**94** d	**95** c	96 d	**97** d	**98** c	**99** a	**100** b
101 c	**102** b	**103** d	**104** d	**105** c	**106** d	**107** d	**108** d	**109** a	**110** c
111 b	**112** b	**113** a	**114**c	**115** d	**116** b	**117** c	**118** b	**119**a	**120** d
121 b	**122** c	**123** b	**124** d	**125** a	**126** b	**127** a	**128** b	**129** b	**130** c
131 d	**132** c	**133** b	**134** c	**135** b	**136** a	**137** d	**138** a	**139**a	**140** d
141 a	**142** b	**143** c	**144** b	**145** d	**146** c	**147** c	**148** b	**149** d	**150** c
151 b	**152** a	**153** d	**154** c	**155** a	**156** b	**157** c	**158** d	**159** c	**160** d
161 d	**162** b	**163** a	**164** a	**165** c	**166** b	**167** c	**168** d	**169**c	**170** c
171 b	**172** d	**173** a	**174** b	**175** c	**176** d	**177** b	**178** c	**179** d	**180** d
181 b	**182** b	**183** c	**184** a	**185** b	**186** d	**187** b	**188** c	**189** a	**190** a
191 b	**192** c	**193** b	**194** a	**195** c	**196** d	**197** b	**198** d	**199** c	**200** a
201 b	**202** c	**203** b	**204** a	**205** c	**206** a	**207** b	**208** c	**209** d	**210** a
211 b	**212** b	**213** b	**214**c	**215** a	**216** d	**217** b	**218** c	**219**c	**220** b

23

Viral Diseases

1 The serotype of aphthovirus causing most outbreaks of FMD in India is

a) A b) O

c) C d) Asia-1

2 The serotype of aphthovirus which is no longer causing FMD outbreak

a) A b) O

c) C d) Asia-1

3 The most common route of transmission of FMD virus in cattle is

a) Ingestion b) Inhalation

c) Cutaneous d) Vector

4 The most common route of transmission of FMD virus in pigs is

a) Ingestion b) Inhalation

c) Cutaneous d) Vector

5 Which of the following species is the most potent excretors of airborne FMD virus?

a) Cattle b) Buffalo

c) Sheep d) Pig

6 Which of the followings is the main site of FMD virus persistence?

a) Buccal mucosa b) Nasopharynx

c) Tonsil d) Nasal mucosa

7 Which of the following species is not susceptible to foot and mouth disease?

a) Elephant b) Deer

c) Horse d) All of the above

8 Appearance of vesicles on the buccal mucosa and feet, long ropy saliva hanging from the mouth along with characteristic smacking of the lips in cattle are the important clinical signs of

a) Vesicular stomatitis b) Vesicular exanthema

c) Foot and mouth disease d) Bovine papillomatosis

9 'Hairy panters' is a common sequel to which disease in cattle?

a) Foot and mouth disease

b) Malignant catarrhal fever

c) Bovine respiratory disease complex

d) Infectious bovine rhinotracheitis

10 Which of the following samples should be collected from the affected animals for the diagnosis of FMD?

a) Oropharyngeal fluid b) Vesicular fluid

c) Affected epithelial tissue d) All of the above

11 'Tiger heart appearance' in calves is the characteristic necropsy finding in

a) Rinderpest b) CBPP

c) FMD d) IBR

12 The most commonly used chemical to inactivate the FMD virus during production of killed vaccine is

a) Formalin

b) Binary ethylene immine (BEI)

c) Glycerol

d) Dolbecco's modified eagle medium

13 Rinderpest virus is antigenically related to virus causing

a) Canine distemper b) PPR in goat

c) Phocine distemper in seal d) All of the above

14 Cattle plague is the synonym of

a) Ephemeral fever b) Blue tongue

c) Rinderpest d) Influenza

15 Bubbly blood-stained salivation in cattle is the characteristic clinical sign in

a) FMD b) Rinderpest

c) BVD-MD d) Vesicular stomatitis

16 Which part of the intestine appears like 'zebra stripes' during PM of cattle died of rinderpest?

a) Colon b) Ileum

c) Jejunum d) Cecum

17 Which type of inclusion bodies are found in tonsils of rinderpest affected cattle?

a) Intranuclear
b) Intracytoplasmic
c) Both a and b
d) No inclusion bodies are found

18 Which of the following disease of cattle is known to be eradicated from the world?

a) Rinderpest
b) Infectious bovine rhinotracheitis
c) Bovine malignant fever
d) Bovine popular stomatitis

19 Goat plague is caused by

a) Picornaviridae
b) Paramyxoviridae
c) Rhabdoviridae
d) Flaviviridae

20 The species most susceptible to PPR virus is

a) Goat
b) Cattle
c) Buffalo
d) Sheep

21 Goats are most susceptible to peste des petits ruminiants at the age of

a) Below 2 months
b) 2-4 months
c) 4 months to 1 year
d) 1-2 year

22 Which form of PPR is most commonly seen in goats?

a) Per-acute
b) Acute
c) Sub-acute
d) Chronic

23 Which form of PPR is most commonly seen in sheep?

a) Per-acute
b) Acute
c) Sub-acute
d) Chronic

24 A kid of 6 month age is presented with a complaint of respiratory distress, diarrhoea, serous nasal and occular discharge with evidence of discrete necrotic lesions on the oral mucosa. Which of the following diseases, the kid is most likely affected with?

a) FMD
b) PPR
c) BVD-MD
d) Vesicular stomatitis

25 Which part of intestine develops a characteristic 'zebra stripes' appearance in a goat died with PPR?

a) Ileo-cecal region
b) Colon
c) Rectum
d) All of the above

26 The causative agent of malignant catarrhal fever (MCF) is

a) α-herpesvirinae b) β-herpesvirinae

c) γ-herpesvirinae d) All of the above

27 At what age, infected sheep mostly excrete ovine herpes virus-2 in their nasal secretions which cause malignant catarrhal fever in cattle?

a) 6-9 months b) Below 6 months

c) 1-2 years d) More than 2 years

28 Which of the following cells are predominantly associated with the vascular lesions in cattle affected with MCF?

a) $CD4^+$ T-lymphocytes b) $CD8^+$ T-lymphocytes

c) B-lymphocytes d) Dendritic cells

29 The most common form of MCF in cattle is

a) Peracute b) Alimentary tract form

c) Head and eye form d) Mild form

30 In head and eye form of MCF, opacity of the cornea commences from

a) Center of cornea b) Periphery of cornea

c) Corneo-scleral junction d) Sclera

31 Which of the following clinical signs is not seen in cattle affected with MCF?

a) Persistence of fever

b) Corneal opacity

c) Ropy and bubbly saliva hanging from the lips

d) None of the above

32 The reservoir host for blue tongue virus is

a) Sheep b) Goat

c) Cattle d) Buffalo

33 Which of the following species acts as amplifier host for blue tongue virus?

a) Pig b) Cattle

c) Bat d) Mongoose

34 The vector commonly responsible for biological transmission of blue tongue virus is

a) Culicoides b) Mosquitoes

c) Stomoxys d) Melophagus

35 Which of the following statements is correct about blue tongue in sheep?
   a) The risk of the disease reduces in dry summer and cold winter
   b) The pathology is attributed to vascular endothelial damage
   c) Merino breed is more susceptible
   d) All of the above

36 Which of the followings is not a clinical manifestation of blue tongue in sheep?
   a) Necrotic ulcers on the lateral aspect of tongue
   b) Dark red to purple band in the skin just above the coronet
   c) Mucopurulent nasal discharge
   d) None of the above

37 Ovine progressive pneumonia is caused by
   a) Pesti virus b) Orbi virus
   c) Lenti virus d) Reovirus

38 Clinical form of Maedi-visna occurs in sheep of age
   a) Below 1 year age b) Below 2 years age
   c) Above 3 years age d) Below 3 years age

39 Hard bag or hard udder condition in sheep is seen in which of the following diseases?
   a) Maedi-visna b) Louping -ill
   c) Jaagsiekte d) Blue tongue

40 Synonym of Maedi-visna in sheep is
   a) Ovine pulmonary adenomatosis
   b) Ovine progressive pneumonia
   c) Ovine enzootic pneumonia
   d) All of the above

41 Synonym of Jaagsiekte in sheep is
   a) Ovine pulmonary adenomatosis
   b) Ovine progressive pneumonia
   c) Ovine enzootic pneumonia
   d) All of the above

42 Ovine pulmonary adenomatosis occurs most commonly in sheep of age
   a) Below 6 months b) 6 months to 1year
   c) 1 to 2 years d) 2 to 4 years

43 Wheel barrow test is applied in sheep for the diagnosis of

a) Maedi-visna b) Jaagsiekte

c) Louping ill d) Orf

44 Jaagsiekte is caused by

a) Retro virus b) Flavi virus

c) Pesti virus d) Orbi virus

45 Louping ill is caused by

a) Retro virus b) Flavi virus

c) Pesti virus d) Orbi virus

46 Bluetongue in sheep is caused by

a) Retro virus b) Flavi virus

c) Pesti virus d) Orbi virus

47 Caprine arthritis encephalitis in goat is caused by

a) Retro virus b) Flavi virus

c) Pesti virus d) Orbi virus

48 Border disease in lambs is caused by

a) Retro virus b) Flavi virus

c) Pesti virus d) Orbi virus

49 Jerky, stiff movements and bounding gait in sheep is the characteristic feature of

a) Blue tongue b) Maedi-visna

c) Louping-ill d) Jaagsiekte

50 Avidin-biotin-complex immunoperoxidase technique can be used for the demonstration of which virus?

a) Louping-ill virus b) Jaagsiekte virus

c) Maedi-visna virus d) Blue tongue virus

51 Hard bag condition of udder in goats occurs in

a) Jaagsiekte b) Blue tongue

c) Caprine arthritis encephalitis d) Contagious ecthyma

52 Which of the following conditions is a clinical manifestation of caprine arthritis encephalitis in goats?

a) Big knee b) Leukoencephalitis

c) Indurative mastitis d) All of the above

53 The causative agent of Contagious ecthyma in young lambs and kids is

a) Cowpox virus b) Parapox virus

c) Capripox virus d) Papilloma virus

54 The causative agent of papillomatosis in young cattle and horses is

a) Cowpox virus b) Parapox virus

c) Capripox virus d) Papilloma virus

55 The causative agent of lumpy skin disease in cattle is

a) Cowpox virus b) Parapox virus

c) Capripox virus d) Papilloma virus

56 Sarcoid in horse is caused by

a) Cowpox virus b) Parapox virus

c) Capripox virus d) Bovine papilloma virus

57 Synonym of contagious ecthyma in sheep is

a) Orf b) Scabby mouth or sore mouth

c) Contagious pustular dermatitis d) All of the above

58 Contagious ecthyma is most commonly occurs in lambs in the group of age

a) Below 3 months b) 3-6 months

c) 6 months to 1 year d) 1-2 year

59 In a sheep affected with contagious ecthyma, the cutaneous lesions develop initially at

a) Oral mucosa b) Nasal mucosa

c) Oral mucocutaneous junction d) Face

60 Appearance of cauliflower like warts in cattle is the characteristic feature

a) Lumpy skin disease b) Bovine papillomatsis

c) Sarcoid d) All of the above

61 Which of the following countries is declared as free from rabies by OIE?

a) Australia b) New Zealand

c) China d) Both (a) and (b)

62 Which strain of rabies virus is considered as vaccine strain?

a) Street virus b) Fixed virus

c) Both of the above d) None of the above

63 The most common mode of transmission of rabies virus is

a) Direct contact b) Ingestion

c) Inhalation d) Bite of an infected animal

64 Which of the following species is considered as subclinical carrier of rabies virus?

a) Bats b) Fox

c) Mongoose d) Dogs

65 Death in rabies commonly occurs due to

a) Damage to brain b) Respiratory paralysis

c) Circulatory failure d) Syncope

66 The yawning movements in cattle is seen in which of following form of rabies?

a) Dumb / Paralytic form b) Furious form

c) Both of the above d) None of the above

67 Which of the following tests is considered as confirmatory for rabies?

a) RIA b) AGID

c) FAT d) IFA

68 Which of the followings is not a pathognomic feature of rabies?

a) Ganglioneuritis b) Suppurative encephalomyelitis

c) Negri bodies d) Babes nodule

69 Negri bodies are most commonly found in which part of the brain in a rabid cattle?

a) Hippocampus b) Purkinje cells of the cerebellum

c) Grey matter of cerebrum d) Hypothalamus

70 Negri bodies are most commonly found in which part of the brain in a rabies virus infected dog?

a) Hippocampus b) Purkinje cells of the cerebellum

c) Grey matter of cerebrum d) Hypothalamus

71 The quarantine period for rabies is

a) 28 days b) 40 days

c) 3 months d) 4-6 months

72 Aujeszky's disease is also known as

a) Viral encephalomyelitis b) Rabies

c) Pseudorabies d) West Nile encephalitis

73 Pseudorabies is caused by

a) Suid herpes virus 1 b) Lyssa virus
c) Retrovirus d) Pestivirus

74 The type of fever seen in bovine ephemeral fever is

a) Intermittent fever b) Remittent fever
c) Biphasic fever d) Persistent fever

75 Bovine ephemeral fever is transmitted by the vector

a) *Culex* spp. b) *Anopheles* spp.
c) *Culicoides* spp. d) All of the above

76 The reservoir host of bovine ephemeral fever is

a) Cattle b) Buffalo
c) Horse d) Pig

77 Which of the following conditions is a feature of bovine ephemeral fever in cattle?

a) Secondary hypocalcemia
b) Serofibrinous polyserositis
c) Accumulation of neutrophils in synovial fluid
d) All of the above

78 Classical swine fever is caused by

a) Pestiviridae b) Asfaviridae
c) Reoviridae d) Retroviridae

79 African swine fever is caused by

a) Pestiviridae b) Asfaviridae
c) Reoviridae d) Retroviridae

80 African horse sickness is caused by

a) Pestiviridae b) Asfaviridae
c) Reoviridae d) Retroviridae

81 Swamp fever in equines is caused by

a) Pestiviridae b) Asfaviridae
c) Reoviridae d) Retroviridae

82 Button shaped ulcer in the colonic mucosa of pigs is the characteristic necropsy finding in

a) Classical swine fever

b) African swine fever

c) Transmissible gastroenteritis of pig

d) PRRS

83 Viral replication in equine infectious anemia occurs in

a) RBCs b) Tissue macrophages

c) Myeloblast d) Lymphocytes

84 Transmission of equine infectious anemia virus in *Stomoxys* fly is

a) Mechanical b) Biological

c) Propagative d) Cyclopropagative

85 Anemia in a horse affected with equine infectious anemia (EIA) occurs due to

a) Intravascular hemolysis by the EIA virus

b) Phagocytosis of RBCs carrying virus-antibody complex on their surface

c) Loss of RBCs due to haemorrhage

d) All of the above

86 Which of the following is a pathological abnormality in equine infectious anemia?

a) Thrombocytopenia

b) Normocytic normochromic anemia

c) Presence of sideroleukocytes

d) All of the above

87 Type of fever seen in equine infectious anemia is

a) Biphasic fever b) Remittent fever

c) Intermittent fever d) Persistent fever

88 Type of fever seen in African horse sickness is

a) Biphasic fever b) Remittent fever

c) Intermittent fever d) Persistent fever

89 African horse sickness may occur in

a) Acute/pulmonary/dunkop form b) Subacute/cardiac/dikkop form

c) Mixed form d) All of the above

90 The most common form of African horse sickness in enzootic area is

a) Dunkop form b) Dikkop form

c) Mixed from d) Mild form

91 Profuse nasal discharge of yellowish serous fluid is found in which form of African horse sickness?

a) Dunkop form b) Dikkop form

c) Mixed from d) Mild form

92 The edema in the head, eyelids, lips and chest is characteristic of which form of African horse sickness?

a) Dunkop form b) Dikkop form

c) Mixed from d) Mild form

93 Bovine spongiform encephalopathy in cattle is caused by

a) Virus b) Cyanobacteria

c) Prion d) Yeast

94 Scrapie in sheep is caused by

a) Virus b) Cyanobacteria

c) Prion d) Yeast

95 Aphthous fever is the synonym of

a) FMD b) Vesicular stomatitis

c) Vesicular exanthema d) Papillomatosis

96 Bovine typhus is also known as

a) FMD b) Rinderpest

c) Q-fever d) Ehrlichiosis

97 Juvenile form of bovine leukosis is seen in calves

a) Below 3 months age b) Below 6 months age

c) 6 months to 1 year age d) Within 10 days of birth

98 Canine distemper in dogs does not occur in which of the following forms?

a) Nervous form b) Digestive form

c) Respiratory form d) None of the above

99 Rubarth's disease is also known as

a) Infectious canine hepatitis b) Blue eye in dogs

c) Contagious hepatitis d) All of the above

100 Canine parvovirus multiplies in which cells of intestine in puppies?

a) Epithelium of villi b) Crypt epithelial cells

c) Peyer's patches d) Submucosal layer of intestine

101 Canine coronavirus multiplies in which cells of intestine in puppies?

a) Epithelium of villi b) Crypt epithelial cells

c) Peyer's patches d) Submucosal layer of intestine

102 Canine rota virus multiplies in which cells of intestine in puppies?

a) Epithelium of villi b) Crypt epithelial cells

c) Peyer's patches d) Submucosal layer of intestine

103 The chief clinical signs of canine parvovirus infection are

a) High fever b) Foul smelling diarrhoea

c) Vomiting d) All of the above

104 The most common type of canine parvovirus causing clinical signs in puppies is

a) CPV-1 b) CPV-2a

c) CPV-2b d) CPV-2c

105 Feline panleukopenia in cats is caused by

a) Retro virus b) Corona virus

c) Parvo virus d) Rota virus

106 Feline rhinotracheitis is caused by

a) Herpes virus b) Adeno virus

c) Corona virus d) Rota virus

107 Pink eye in equines is also known as

a) Equine infectious anemia b) Equine viral arteritis

c) Equine encephalomyelitis d) African horse sickness

108 Fowl pox in domestic fowl is caused by

a) Herpes virus b) Paramyxo virus

c) Birna virus d) Avipox virus

109 Marek's disease in poultry is caused by

a) Herpes virus b) Paramyxo virus

c) Birna virus d) Avipox virus

110 Newcastle disease in chicks is caused by

a) Herpes virus b) Paramyxo virus
c) Birna virus d) Avipox virus

111 Infectious laryngotracheitis in chicken is caused by

a) Herpes virus b) Paramyxo virus
c) Birna virus d) Avipox virus

112 Infectious bronchitis in chicks is caused by

a) Circo virus b) Corona virus
c) Retro virus d) Birna virus

113 Infectious bursal disease is caused by

a) Circo virus b) Corona virus
c) Retro virus d) Birna virus

114 Lymphoid leukosis in chicken is caused by

a) Circo virus b) Corona virus
c) Retro virus d) Birna virus

115 Chicken infectious anemia is caused by

a) Circo virus b) Corona virus
c) Retro virus d) Birna virus

116 Fowl pox is characterized by

a) Nodular lesions on featherless part
b) Necrotic lesions on the mucosa
c) Chronic emaciation
d) All of the above

117 Fowl pox in chicken may occur in which of the following forms?

a) Cutaneous form b) Diphtheritic form
c) Wet pox d) All of the above

118 Diphtheritic form of fowl pox is characterized by

a) Necrotic lesions in the oral and respiratory mucosa
b) Coughing
c) Both (a) and (b)
d) Nodules on the featherless part

119 Bollinger bodies is the characteristic histological finding in which disease in poultry?

a) Fowl pox
b) Marek's disease
c) Avian influenza
d) Fowl cholera

120 Greenish diarrhoea in chicken is found in which of the following diseases?

a) Fowl pox
b) Marek's disease
c) Avian influenza
d) Lymphoid leukosis

121 Classical form of marek's disease is characterized by

a) Unilateral/bilateral paralysis
b) Tumors in the visceral organs
c) Both of the above
d) None of the above

122 Acute form of Marek's disease is characterized by

a) Unilateral/bilateral paralysis
b) Tumors in the visceral organs
c) Both of the above
d) None of the above

123 Tumors in Marek's disease is mainly comprise of

a) T lymphocytes
b) B lymphocytes
c) Epithelial cells
d) Basal cells of skin

124 Tumors in lymphoid leukosis in birds is mainly comprise of

a) T lymphocytes
b) B lymphocytes
c) Epithelial cells
d) Basal cells of skin

125 Big liver disease in birds is also known as

a) Lymphoid leukosis
b) Visceral lymphomatosis
c) Avian leukosis
d) All of the above

126 Vertical transmission is seen in which of the following diseases?

a) Lymphoid leukosis
b) Marek's disease
c) Infectious bursal disease
d) Fowl pox

127 COFAL test is associated with which of the following diseases?

a) Chicken infectious anemia
b) Marek's disease
c) Lymphoid leukosis
d) Fowl pox

128 Which of the followings is a highly contagious, immunosuppressive disease of chicken?

a) MD
b) IBD
c) RD
d) Fowl pox

129 Ecchymotic hemorrhage at the junction of gizzard and proventriculus, pale appearance of kidney with urate deposits and enlargement of bursa are the characteristic PM findings of which disease?

a) RD b) MD

c) IBD d) Chicken infectious anemia

130 Pin-point hemorrhages at the apex of proventriculus is found in

a) RD b) MD

c) IBD d) Chicken infectious anemia

131 F and LaSota strain belong to which pathotype of Newcastle disease virus

a) Velogenic b) Lentogenic

c) Mesogenic d) All of the above

132 R_2B strain belongs to which pathotype of Newcastle disease virus

a) Velogenic b) Lentogenic

c) Mesogenic d) All of the above

133 Edema and cyanotic swelling of comb, wattle and eyelids in chicken is found in

a) Fowl pox b) Avian influenza

c) Lymphoid leukosis d) Infectious bronchitis

134 Which species of domestic birds is most susceptible to avian influenza?

a) Chicken b) Turkey

c) Quail d) Guinea fowl

135 The incubation period of avian influenza virus is

a) Few hours to 3 days b) 1-7 days

c) 7-14 days d) More than 14 days

136 Which of the following species is considered as the mixing vessel for avian and mammalian influenza virus?

a) Cattle b) Buffalo

c) Pig d) Horse

137 Avian encephalomyelitis is also known as

a) Avian plague b) White comb disease

c) Split leg disease d) Epidemic tremor

138 Death of chicks affected with avian encephalomyelitis is mainly due to

a) Asphyxia b) Hemorrhage

c) Tampling by fellow pen-mates d) Inanition

139 Which of the followings is not a clinical feature of infectious laryngotracheitis in birds?

a) Gasping

b) Conjunctivitis

c) Expectoration of exudates with blood

d) None of the above

140 Chicken infectious anemia is characterized by

a) Aplastic anemia | b) Generalized lymphoid atrophy

c) Immunosuppression | d) All of the above

141 A week-old chick should be vaccinated with which strain of ranikhet disease virus?

a) F | b) R_2B

c) LaSota | d) Roakin

142 The route of RD vaccination in chicks is

a) Intranasal | b) Intraocular

c) Subcutaneous | d) Both a and b

143 The dose of rabies vaccine in all animals is

a) 0.5 ml | b) 1 ml

c) 2 ml | d) 5 ml

144 In India, the trivalent vaccine for cats includes which of the following diseases?

a) Feline rhinotracheitis | b) Feline calici virus infection

c) Feline panleukopenia | d) All of the above

145 The type of vaccine in commonly used rabies vaccine for post-exposure prophylaxis?

a) Inactivated tissue culture | b) Live attenuated

c) Bivalent vaccine | d) Multivalent vaccine

Answer Key

1 b	**2** c	**3** b	**4** a	**5** d	**6** b	**7** c	**8** c	**9** a	**10** d
11 c	**12** b	**13** d	**14** c	**15** b	**16** a	**17** c	**18** a	**19** b	**20** a
21 c	**22** b	**23** c	**24** b	**25** d	**26** c	**27** a	**28** b	**29** c	**30** c
31 d	**32** c	**33** b	**34** a	**35** d	36 d	**37** c	**38** c	**39** a	**40** b
41 a	**42** d	**43** b	**44** a	**45** b	**46** d	**47** a	**48** c	**49** c	**50** a
51 c	**52** d	**53** c	**54** d	**55** c	**56** d	**57** d	**58** b	**59** c	**60** b
61 d	**62** b	**63** d	**64** a	**65** b	**66** b	**67** c	**68** b	**69** b	**70** a
71 d	**72** c	**73** a	**74** c	**75** d	**76** a	**77** d	**78** a	**79** b	**80** c
81 d	**82** a	**83** b	**84** a	**85** b	**86** d	**87** c	**88** c	**89** d	**90** b
91 a	**92** b	**93** c	**94** c	**95** a	**96** b	**97** b	**98** d	**99** d	**100** b
101 a	**102** a	**103** d	**104** c	**105** c	**106** a	**107** b	**108** d	**109** a	**110** b
111 a	**112** b	**113** d	**114** c	**115** a	**116** d	**117** d	**118** c	**119**a	**120** b
121 a	**122** b	**123** a	**124** b	**125** d	**126** a	**127** a	**128** b	**129** c	**130** a
131 b	**132** c	**133** b	**134**b	**135** a	**136** c	**137** d	**138** c	**139**d	**140** d
141 c	**142** d	**143** b	**144**d	**145** a					

24

Parasitic Diseases

1 The causative agent of red water fever in cattle is

a) *Babesia bigemina* b) *Leptospira interrogans*

c) *Theileria annulata* d) *Theileria parva*

2 Pipe stem faeces in bovines is caused by

a) *Babesia bigemina* b) *Babesia bovis*

c) *Babesia divergens* d) All of the above

3 Which stage of the parasite is found in blood smear of cattle affected with babesiosis?

a) Schizont b) Sporozoites

c) Ray bodies d) Merozoites

4 Which of the following clinical signs is not seen in animals affected with babesiosis?

a) High temperature b) Hematuria

c) Anemia d) Jaundice

5 The drug of choice for babesiosis is

a) Buparvaquone b) Oxytetracycline

c) Diminazene aceturate d) Ivermectin

6 The dose rate of diminazene aceturate for the treatment of babesiosis in dog is

a) 2.5 mg/kg b) 3.5 mg/kg

c) 4.5 mg/kg d) 5 mg/kg

7 Incidence of babesiosis in farm animals is more during

a) Summer b) Rainy

c) Winter d) Both (a) and (b)

8 Vector responsible for transmission of canine babesiosis is

a) *Rhipicephalus sanguineus* b) *Rhipicephalus everti*

c) *Rhipicephalus bursa* d) *Boophilus microplus*

9 Which of the following *babesia spp.* has classical maltese cross appearance inside the erythrocytes?

a) *B. bovis* b) *B. bigemina*

c) *B. caballi* d) *B. equi*

10 Cerebral babesiosis in cattle is caused by

a) *B. bovis* b) *B. bigemina*

c) *B. divergens* d) *B. major*

11 Pirodog is a vaccine against which disease?

a) Babesiosis b) Anaplasmosis

c) Theileriosis d) Ehrlichiosis

12 East coast fever is caused by

a) *Theileria sergenti* b) *Theileria parva*

c) *Theileria annulata* d) *Theileria hirci*

13 Mediterranean coast fever is caused by

a) *Theileria sergenti* b) *Theileria parva*

c) *Theileria annulata* d) *Theileria hirci*

14 Oriental theileriosis in bovines is caused by

a) *Theileria orientalis* b) *Theileria parva*

c) *Theileria annulata* d) *Theileria hirci*

15 Benign ovine theileriosis is caused by

a) *Theileria orientalis* b) *Theileria parva*

c) *Theileria ovis* d) *Theileria hirci*

16 Malignant ovine theileriosis is caused by

a) *Theileria orientalis* b) *Theileria parva*

c) *Theileria ovis* d) *Theileria hirci*

17 Cerebral theileriosis in cattle is caused by

a) *Theileria annulata* b) *Theileria parva*

c) *Theileria orientalis* d) *Theileria sergenti*

18 The vector of East coast fever is

a) *Rhipicephalus appendiculatus*

b) *Hyalomma* spp.

c) *Haemaphysalis* spp.

d) *Amblyomma* spp.

19 The vector of bovine tropical theileriosis is

a) *Rhipicephalus appendiculatus*

b) *Hyalomma* spp.

c) *Haemaphysalis* spp.

d) *Amblyomma* spp.

20 The stage of theileria organism which infect the erythrocytes is

a) Schizont b) Kochs blue bodies

c) Piroplasm d) Merozoite

21 Punched out necrotic ulcers in the abomasum is the pathognomic lesions of which disease in calves?

a) Theileriosis b) Babesiosis

c) Anaplasmosis d) Trypanosomosis

22 In *Theileria annulata* infection, schizont is formed mostly in which cells?

a) Lymphocyte b) Neutrophill

c) Macrophages d) Basophils

23 The dose of buparvaquone for the treatment of theileriosis is

a) 2.5 mg/kg b) 5 mg/kg

c) 10 mg/kg d) 20 mg/kg

24 In which of the following disease, anemia is not a significant clinical finding?

a) Tropical theileriosis b) Anaplasmosis

c) East coast fever d) Babesiosis

25 Development of pulmonary edema in cattle is found in which of the following parasitic infections?

a) *Theileria annulata* b) *Theileria parva*

c) *Theileria orientalis* d) *Theileria sergenti*

26 Most commonly used vaccine for theileriosis is

a) Live attenuated cell culture vaccine b) Inactivated vaccine

c) Recombinant vaccine d) None of the above

27 Nagana disease or African trypanosomosis is caused by

a) *Trypanosoma evansi* b) *Trypanosoma congolense*

c) *Trypanosoma cruzi* d) *Trypanosoma theileri*

28 Chagas disease is caused by

a) *Trypanosoma evansi* b) *Trypanosoma congolense*

c) *Trypanosoma cruzi* d) *Trypanosoma theileri*

29 Surra in camel is caused by

a) *Trypanosoma evansi* b) *Trypanosoma congolense*

c) *Trypanosoma cruzi* d) *Trypanosoma theileri*

30 Dourine in horse is caused by

a) *Trypanosoma evansi* b) *Trypanosoma congolense*

c) *Trypanosoma cruzi* d) *Trypanosoma equiperdum*

31 The main vector for transmission of African trypanosomosis is

a) *Glossina* spp. b) *Tabanus* spp.

c) *Rhodinus* spp. d) *Triatoma* spp.

32 The main vector responsible for transmission of surra in India is

a) *Glossina* spp. b) *Tabanus* spp.

c) *Rhodinus* spp. d) *Triatoma* spp.

33 Dourine is transmitted by

a) Biting flies b) Veneral transmission

c) Direct contact d) Ticks

34 Which of the followings is preferred for the detection of trypanosoma organism?

a) Thin blood smear b) Thick blood smear

c) Plasma d) Lymph node aspirate

35 "Silver dollar spot" on body and neck is the characteristic finding of

a) Cutaneous leishmaniasis b) Bovine lymphosarcoma

c) Dourine d) Lumpy skin disease

36 Which of the following tests can be used for the detection of trypanosomosis?

a) Stilbamidine test b) Formal gel tube test

c) Mercuric chloride test d) All of the above

37 The dose of quinapyramine for the treatment of trypanosomosis is

a) 5 mg/kg b) 10 mg/kg

c) 20 mg/kg d) 50 mg/kg

38 Rat tail appearance in cattle may be seen in which of the following protozoal diseases?

a) Cutaneous leishmaniasis b) Coccidiosis

c) Sarcocystosis d) Neosporosis

39 Which of the following species act as the definitive host for *Sarcocystis* spp.?

a) Cattle b) Dog

c) Cat d) Both (b) and (c)

40 Which of the following species act as the intermediate host for *Sarcocystis* spp.?

a) Cattle b) Sheep

c) Pig d) All of the above

41 Definitive host of *Sarcocystis* acquire the infection through

a) Feeding of raw meat

b) Ingestion of feed contaminated with faeces

c) Both of the above

d) None of the above

42 Intermediate host of *Sarcocystis* acquire the infection through

a) Feeding of raw meat

b) Ingestion of feed contaminated with faeces

c) Both of the above

d) None of the above

43 The stage of *Sarcocystis* which is infective to dog and cat is

a) Bradyzoites b) Tachyzoites

c) Macrogametes d) Microgametes

44 The major route of *Neospora caninum* transmission in cattle is

a) Horizontal transmission

b) Vertical transmission

c) Ingestion of faeces contaminated with dog faeces

d) None of the above

45 The definitive host of *Neospora caninum* is

a) Cattle b) Buffalo

c) Dog d) Cat

46 Which of the following protozoal organisms is associated with endemic and epidemic abortion in cattle?

a) *Sarcocystis* b) *Neospora*

c) *Trypanosoma* d) *Eimeria*

47 Which of the following organisms does not cause diarrhoea in young ruminants?

a) Coccidia b) Giardia

c) Cryptosporidium d) Neospora

48 Equine protozoal myeloencephalitis (EPM) is caused by

a) *Trypanosoma evansi* b) *Sarcocystis neurona*

c) *Babesia equi* d) *Theileria equi*

49 The definitive host of *Toxoplasma gondii* is

a) Cat b) Dog

c) Sheep d) Pig

50 The infective stage of *Toxoplasma* found in cat faeces is

a) Bradyzoites b) Tachyzoites

c) Oocysts d) Macrogamots

51 Hepatic coccidiosis in rabbit is caused by

a) *Eimeria tenella* b) *Eimeria necatrix*

c) *Eimeria stiedae* d) *Eimeria acervulina*

52 Caecal coccidiosis in poultry birds is caused by

a) *Eimeria tenella* b) *Eimeria necatrix*

c) *Eimeria stiedae* d) *Eimeria acervulina*

53 Rectal coccidiosis in poultry birds is caused by

a) *Eimeria tenella* b) *Eimeria brunetti*

c) *Eimeria stiedae* d) *Eimeria acervulina*

54 Intestinal coccidiosis in poultry birds is caused by

a) *Eimeria tenella* b) *Eimeria brunetti*

c) *Eimeria stiedae* d) *Eimeria necatrix*

55 Coccidia organisms are

a) Host specific b) Organ specific

c) Cell specific d) All of the above

56 Caecal core in chicken is the characteristic necropsy finding of

a) *Eimeria necatrix* infection b) *Eimeria tenella* infection

c) *Eimeria acervulina* infection d) *Eimeria brunetti* infection

57 The most pathogenic *Eimeria* spp. in cattle and buffaloes is

a) *E. bovis* b) *E. zuernii*

c) *E. auburnensis* d) *E. ellipsoidalis*

58 The most pathogenic *Eimeria* spp. in poultry is

a) *Eimeria tenella* b) *Eimeria brunetti*

c) *Eimeria acervulina* d) *E. bovis*

59 The dose of amprolium for the treatment of coccidiosis in calves is

a) 5 mg/kg b) 10 mg/kg

c) 15 mg/kg d) 20 mg/kg

60 In ruminants, clinically affected with coccidiosis, the oocyst count in faeces should be

a) ≥ 1000 oocyst/g b) ≥ 2000 oocyst/g

c) ≥ 3000 oocyst/g d) ≥ 5000 oocyst/g

61 Which of the following drugs is contraindicated for the treatment of coccidiosis

a) Monensin b) Decoquinate

c) Dexamethasone d) Toltrazuril

62 Which vitamin supplementation is advisable during the treatment of coccidiosis?

a) Vit. A b) Vit. E

c) Vit. C d) All of the above

63 Visceral leishmanosis is caused by

a) *Leishmania donovani* b) *Leishmania tropica*

c) *Leishmania major* d) *Leishmania Mexicana*

64 Cutaneous leishmanosis is caused by

a) *Leishmania donovani* b) *Leishmania tropica*

c) *Leishmania infantum* d) *Leishmania braziliensis*

65 Muco-cutaneous leishmanosis is caused by

a) *Leishmania donovani* b) *Leishmania tropica*

c) *Leishmania infantum* d) *Leishmania braziliensis*

66 The form of leishmania found in vertebrate host is

a) Amastigote b) Promastigote

c) Both of the above d) None of the above

67 The form of leishmania found in sand fly vector is

a) Amastigote b) Promastigote

c) Both of the above d) None of the above

68 Leishmanosis does not occur in

a) Dog b) Human

c) Cattle d) Rodents

69 Montenegro test is applied for the diagnosis of

a) Toxoplasmosis b) Neosporosis

c) Trypanosomosis d) Leishmanosis

70 The most serious form of leishmanosis in dogs is

a) Visceral leishmanosis b) Moist-cutaneous leishmanosis

c) Dry-cutaneous leishmanosis d) Muco-cutaneous leishmanosis

71 Self-cure phenomenon is seen by

a) *Ostertagia circumcincta* b) *Haemonchus contortus*

c) *Haemonchus placei* d) *Trichostrongylus axei*

72 *Haemonchus placei* is most commonly found in

a) Sheep b) Goat

c) Cattle d) Horse

73 Which of the followings is known as babrber's pole worm?

a) *Haemonchus contortus* b) *Ostertagia circumcincta*

c) *Trichostrongylus axei* d) *Ostertagia ostertagi*

74 Haemonchosis in calves is characterized clinically by

a) Anemia b) Anasarca

c) Wasting d) All of the above

75 Definitive host of *Bunostomum trigonocephalum* is

a) Cattle b) Sheep

c) Goat d) Pig

76 Definitive host of *Bunostomum phlebotomum* is

a) Cattle b) Sheep

c) Goat d) Pig

77 Which of the following organisms is responsible for occurrence of GID in sheep?

a) *Taenia ovis* b) *Taenia pisiformis*

c) *Taenia multiceps* d) *Taenia taniaformis*

78 Which of the following organisms is responsible for development of lung cyst in cattle?

a) *Taenia saginatta* b) *Echinococcus granulosus*

c) *Anoplocephala perfoliata* d) *Moniezia benedeni*

79 Casoni's intracutaneous test is done for the diagnosis of

a) Neurocysticercosis b) GID

c) False GID d) Echinococcosis

80 Which of the following parasites is responsible for anal pruritus in dog?

a) *Dipylidium caninum* b) *Diphyllobothrium latum*

c) *Mesocestoides lineatum* d) *Dioctophyma renale*

81 Which of the following parasitic infections occurs in dogs due to swallowing of infected cat flea?

a) *Dioctophyma renale* b) *Dipylidium caninum*

c) *Ancylostoma caninum* d) *Toxocara canis*

82 The drug of choice for cestodal infection in animals is

a) Ivermectin b) Doramectin

c) Praziquantel d) Closantel

83 Which of the following parasites causes verminous bronchitis in cattle?

a) *Dictyocaulus filaria* b) *Dictyocaulus viviparus*

c) *Protostrongylus rufescens* d) *Mullerius capillaris*

84 Which of the following drugs is commonly used as prophylaxis for heart worm disease in dogs?

a) Diethylcarbamazine b) Levamisole

c) Albendazole d) Oxyclozanide

85 Kumri in horses is caused by

a) *Anoplocephala perfoliata* b) *Strongylus vulgaris*

c) *Setaria edentata* d) *Trypanosoma evansi*

86 Eye worm of cattle is

a) *Thelazia rhodesi* b) *Thelazia capillata*

c) *Thelazia lacrymalis* d) *Thelazia califoriensis*

87 Kidney worm of swine is

a) *Dioctophyma renale* b) *Setaria edentata*

c) *Stephanurus dentatus* d) *Diphyllobothrium latum*

88 Passing of mud-coloured faeces in calves is found in infection with

a) *Toxocara vitulorum* b) *Fasciola hepatica*

c) *Pramphistomum cervi* d) *Gigantocotyl explanatum*

89 Which of the following parasites causes vesceral larva migrans in dogs?

a) *Ancylostoma caninum* b) *Toxocara canis*

c) *Dioctophyma renale* d) *Dipylidium caninum*

90 Which parasite causes rat tail condition in horse?

a) *Strongylus vulgaris* b) *Parascaris equorum*

c) *Strongyloides westeri* d) *Oxyuris equi*

91 Verminous aneurysm in horse is caused by

a) *Strongylus vulgaris* b) *Parascaris equorum*

c) *Strongyloides westeri* d) *Oxyuris equi*

92 Which of the following parasite is associated with pimply gut condition in sheep?

a) *Oesophagostomum columbianum* b) *Ostertagia ostertagii*

c) *Strongyloides papillosus* d) *Strongyloides ransomi*

93 Pipe stem liver condition in cattle is seen in

a) Ascariasis b) Fasciolosis

c) Haemonchosis d) Amphistomosis

94 Biliary amphistomosis in buffalo is caused by

a) *Paramphistomum cervi* b) *Gastrothylax crumenifer*

c) *Gigantococtyl explanatum* d) *Gastrodiscoides hominis*

95 Napoleon's hat shaped egg is found in

a) *Dicrocoelium dendriticum* b) *Schistosoma nasalis*

c) *Paragonimus westermanii* d) *Clonorchis sinensis*

96 The drug of choice for fasciolosis is

a) Triclabendazole b) Oxyclozanide

c) Closantel d) Pyrantel pamoate

97 Snoring disease in cattle is caused by which parasite?

a) *Schistosoma nasalis* b) *Paragonimus westermanii*

c) *Dictyocaulus viviparus* d) *Echinococcus granulosus*

98 The larva of which of the following fly cause 'snotty nose' condition or 'False GID' in sheep?

a) *Hypoderma crossi* b) *Oestrus ovis*

c) *Stomoxys calcitrans* d) *Glossina palpalis*

99 Morocco leather appearance of gastric mucosa is seen in

a) Fasciolosis b) Amphistomosis

c) Oestertagiosis d) Echinococcosis

100 Milk spot in liver of pig is seen due to infection with

a) *Fasciola hepatica* b) *Ascaris suum*

c) *Stephanurus dentatus* d) *Diphyllobothrium latum*

101 Black head disease in chicken is caused by

a) *Davainea proglottina* b) *Histomonas meleagridis*

c) *Railietina tetragona* d) *Cotugnia digonopora*

102 Appearance of sulphur yellow droopings of turkey occurs due to infection with

a) *Davainea proglottina* b) *Histomonas meleagridis*

c) *Railietina tetragona* d) *Cotugnia digonopora*

103 Which of the followings is known as red mites of poultry?

a) *Cnemidocoptes mutans* b) *Cnemidocoptes gallinae*

c) *Dermanyssus gallinae* d) *Ornithonyssus bursa*

104 Depluming itch in fowl is caused by

a) *Cnemidocoptes mutans* b) *Cnemidocoptes gallinae*

c) *Dermanyssus gallinae* d) *Ornithonyssus bursa*

105 Scaly leg in fowl is caused by

a) *Cnemidocoptes mutans* b) *Cnemidocoptes gallinae*

c) *Dermanyssus gallinae* d) *Ornithonyssus bursa*

106 Auricular mange in dog is caused by

a) Psoroptes b) Sarcoptes

c) Otodectes d) All of the above

107 Sarcoptes is mainly found in

a) Body parts having less or no hair

b) Body parts well covered with hairs

c) Hair follicle

d) None of the above

108 Which of the following drugs should not be used for the treatment of canine demodicosis?

a) Fluralaner b) Closantel

c) Prednisolone d) All of the above

109 Summer sore is caused by

a) Oestertagiasis b) Filariasis

c) Ascariasis d) Habronemiasis

110 The predilection site of *Dirofilarial immitis* in dog is

a) Anterior mesenteric artery b) Right ventricle

c) Right auricle d) Carotid artery

111 Which of the followings should be given in combination with amprolium for the treatment of coccidiosis in poultry?

a) Vitamin B complex b) Folic acid

c) Cholecalciferol d) Biotin

112 The immunostimulant dose of levamisole is

a) 2.5 mg/kg b) 5 mg/kg

c) 7.5 mg/kg d) 10 mg/kg

113 Which of the following parasite is associated with development of neurocysticercosis in human?

a) *Taenia saginatta* b) *Taenia solium*

c) *Taenia multiceps* d) *Taenia serialis*

114 Bottle jaw condition is seen in

a) Haemonchosis b) Fasciolosis

c) Paramphistomosis d) All of the above

115 Modified knott test is used for the detection of

a) *Setaria digitata* b) *Dirofilaria immitis*

c) *Stephanurus dentatus* d) *Sarcocystis neurona*

116 Sabin fieldman dye test used for the diagnosis of

a) Echinococcosis b) Leishmaniosis

c) Toxoplasmosis d) Cryptosporidiosis

117 Cutaneous larva migrans is caused due to migration of

a) Toxocara larva b) Ancylostoma larva

c) Strongyle larva d) Haemonchus larva

118 Cucumber seed shaped gravid segment in the faeces of dogs is the characteristic of

a) *Echinococcus granulosus* b) *Dipylidium caninum*

c) *Diphyllobothrium latum* d) *Taenia hydatigena*

119 Hump sore is caused by

a) *Habronema majus* b) *Stephanofilaria zaheri*

c) *Stephanofilaria assamensis* d) *Stephanofilaria stelesi*

120 Ear sore in buffalo is caused by

a) *Habronema megastoma* b) *Stephanofilaria zaheri*

c) *Stephanofilaria assamensis* d) *Stephanofilaria stelesi*

121 Enzootic cerebrospinal nematodiasis is caused by

a) *Thelazia rhodesi* b) *Trichinella spiralis*

c) *Capillaria annulata* d) *Setaria digitata*

122 Tick GARD vaccine is used against which of the following tick?

a) *Otobius megnini* b) *Boophilus micropus*

c) *Rhipicephalus sanguineus* d) *Ornithodoros moubata*

123 Which of the following bacteria is used for the biological control of ticks?

a) *Bacillus thuringiensis* b) *Aeromonas hydrophila*

c) *Vibrio parahaemolyticus* d) *Pseudomonas aeruginosa*

124 The dose of ivermectin in rabbit is

a) 100 mcg/kg b) 200 mcg/kg

c) 400 mcg/kg d) 500 mcg/kg

125 Amitraz should be used for the treatment of canine demodicosis at a concentration of

a) 0.25% b) 0.025%

c) 0.05% d) 0.5%

Answer Key

1 a	**2** c	**3** b	**4** b	**5** c	**6** b	**7** d	**8** a	**9** d	**10** b
11 a	**12** b	**13** c	**14** a	**15** c	**16** d	**17** b	**18** a	**19** b	**20** d
21 a	**22** c	**23** a	**24** c	**25** b	**26** a	**27** b	**28** c	**29** a	**30** d
31 a	**32** b	**33** b	**34** b	**35** c	**36** d	**37** a	**38** c	**39** d	**40** d
41 a	**42** b	**43** a	**44** b	**45** c	**46** b	**47** d	**48** b	**49** a	**50** c
51 c	**52** a	**53** b	**54** d	**55** d	**56** b	**57** b	**58** a	**59** b	**60** d
61 c	**62** d	**63** a	**64** b	**65** d	**66** a	**67** b	**68** c	**69** d	**70** a
71 b	**72** c	**73** a	**74** d	**75** b	**76** a	**77** c	**78** b	**79** d	**80** a
81 b	**82** c	**83** b	**84** a	**85** c	**86** a	**87** c	**88** a	**89** b	**90** d
91 a	**92** a	**93** b	**94** c	**95** b	**96** a	**97** a	**98** b	**99** c	**100** a
101 b	**102** b	**103** c	**104** b	**105** a	**106** c	**107** a	**108** c	**109** d	**110** b
111 a	**112** a	**113** b	**114** d	**115** b	**116** c	**117** b	**118** b	**119** c	**120** b
121 d	**122** b	**123** a	**124** c	**125** b					

25

Epidemiology

1 Study of distribution of diseases and the factors determining its distribution in a population is known as

a) Ethology b) Epidemiology

c) Ecology d) Etiology

2 The primary objective of epidemiology is

a) To identify the etiology and risk factors associated with the disease

b) To determine pathogen distribution, the virulency basis of the disease

c) To develop suitable preventive measures to control

d) All of the above

3 The word 'epidemiology' is derived from

a) Latin word b) Greek word

c) Both of the above d) None of the above

4 Which of the followings involves analysis of observations using appropriate statistical tools

a) Descriptive epidemiology b) Experimental epidemiology

c) Analytical epidemiology d) Theoretical epidemiology

5 Which of the followings involves the field and clinical trial for the study of a disease

a) Descriptive epidemiology b) Experimental epidemiology

c) Analytical epidemiology d) Theoretical epidemiology

6 Which of the followings uses mathematical models resembling natural disease patterns

a) Descriptive epidemiology b) Experimental epidemiology

c) Analytical epidemiology d) Theoretical epidemiology

7 Which of the followings involves observation and recording of diseases in animals and possible causal factors

a) Descriptive epidemiology b) Experimental epidemiology

c) Analytical epidemiology d) Theoretical epidemiology

8 Which of the followings is associated with generation of hypothesis

a) Descriptive epidemiology b) Experimental epidemiology

c) Analytical epidemiology d) Theoretical epidemiology

9 Outbreak of disease in animal population is known as

a) Epidemic b) Endemic

c) Epizootic d) Enzootic

10 Outbreak of disease in avian population is known as

a) Epidemic b) Endemic

c) Epizootic d) Epornitics

11 Occurrence of a disease in a population at a level higher than usual is known as

a) Epidemic b) Endemic

c) Sporadic d) Pandemic

12 Constant presence of a disease in a population is known as

a) Epidemic b) Endemic

c) Sporadic d) Pandemic

13 Widespread occurrence of a disease involving many countries and continent is called as

a) Epidemic b) Endemic

c) Sporadic d) Pandemic

14 Infrequent and haphazard occurrence of a disease in known as

a) Epidemic b) Endemic

c) Sporadic d) Pandemic

15 The characteristic disease pattern in epidemic is

a) Temporal clustering only

b) Spatial clustering only

c) Both temporal and spatial clustering

d) None of the above

16 The characteristic pattern in endemic disease is

a) Temporal clustering only

b) Spatial clustering only

c) Both temporal and spatial clustering

d) None of the above

17 The characteristic pattern in pandemic disease is

a) Temporal clustering only

b) Spatial clustering only

c) Both temporal and spatial clustering

d) None of the above

18 The characteristic pattern in sporadic disease is

a) Temporal clustering only

b) Spatial clustering only

c) Both temporal and spatial clustering

d) None of the above

19 Foot and Mouth disease is an example of

a) Epidemic disease b) Endemic disease

c) Sporadic disease d) Pandemic disease

20 Anthrax is an example of _______ disease

a) Epidemic b) Endemic

c) Sporadic d) Pandemic

21 Avian influenza is an example of ________ disease

a) Epidemic b) Endemic

c) Sporadic d) Pandemic

22 The disease of foreign origin that enters new geographical area either through migration of animals or through import of animal product is known as

a) Epidemic b) Endemic

c) Exotic d) Exzootic

23 Disease that has been localized to particular geographical area is known as

a) Epidemic b) Endemic

c) Exotic d) Exzootic

24 Which of the followings is considered as a determinant of a disease

a) Breed b) Virus

c) Water d) All of the above

25 Minimum amount of infectious agent required to initiate a the disease process is called

a) Virulency b) Infectivity

c) Pathogenicity d) Latency

26 Quality of disease induced by the organism is called as

a) Virulency b) Infectivity

c) Pathogenicity d) Latency

27 Ability of an organism to produce disease in a host in terms of severity is known as

a) Virulency b) Infectivity

c) Pathogenicity d) Latency

28 Ability of an organism to remain quiescent in a host is known as

a) Virulency b) Infectivity

c) Pathogenicity d) Latency

29 The time period between exposure to an agent and appearance of clinical signs is

a) Incubation period b) Prepatent period

c) Generation time d) Extrinsic incubation period

30 The time period between infection and shedding of organism from the host is

a) Incubation period b) Prepatent period

c) Generation time d) Extrinsic incubation period

31 The time period between infection and maximum infectiousness is

a) Incubation period b) Prepatent period

c) Generation time d) Extrinsic incubation period

32 The time period between infection and availability of agent in arthropod vectors is

a) Incubation period b) Prepatent period

c) Generation time d) Extrinsic incubation period

33 The carrier who sheds the organism during incubation period of the disease is

a) Convalescent carrier b) Incubatory carrier

c) Healthy carrier d) Temporary carrier

34 The carrier who sheds the organism during recovery stage of the disease is

a) Convalescent carrier b) Incubatory carrier

c) Healthy carrier d) Temporary carrier

35 The carrier who sheds the organism for short period of time is

a) Convalescent carrier b) Incubatory carrier

c) Healthy carrier d) Temporary carrier

36 The cause without which the disease cannot occur is known as

a) Necessary cause b) Sufficient cause

c) Both of the above d) None of the above

37 The cause which produces the disease only in presence of the necessary cause is called as

a) Necessary cause b) Sufficient cause

c) Both of the above d) None of the above

38 The factor that is associated with the definitive onset of disease process is

a) Predisposing factor b) Enabling factor

c) Precipitating factor d) Reinforcing factor

39 The factor that enhances the susceptibility in the host

a) Predisposing factor b) Enabling factor

c) Precipitating factor d) Reinforcing factor

40 The factors that ease the manifestation of a disease

a) Predisposing factor b) Enabling factor

c) Precipitating factor d) Reinforcing factor

41 The factor that tends to aggravate the presence of a disease

a) Predisposing factor b) Enabling factor

c) Precipitating factor d) Reinforcing factor

42 Immune status of the host is an example of

a) Predisposing factor b) Enabling factor

c) Precipitating factor d) Reinforcing factor

43 Repeated exposure to an infectious agent in the absence of immune response is an example of

a) Predisposing factor b) Enabling factor

c) Precipitating factor d) Reinforcing factor

44 The number of new cases arising in a population in a given period of time is known as

a) Attack rate b) Prevalence

c) Incidence d) Case fatality rate

45 The ability of a disease condition to cause death of affected individuals in a specified time is known as

a) Attack rate b) Prevalence

c) Incidence d) Case fatality rate

46 Incidence is a

a) Proportion b) Rate

c) Percentage d) Ratio

47 Prevalence is a

a) Proportion b) Rate

c) Percentage d) Ratio

48 Reduction in the morbidity and mortality from the disease is known as

a) Prevention b) Control

c) Eradication d) Elimination

49 Reduction in the incidence of the disease below the level achieved by control is called as

a) Prevention b) Control

c) Eradication d) Elimination

50 Regional extinction of an infectious agent is known as

a) Prevention b) Control

c) Eradication d) Elimination

51 Type of prevention which involves detection and prompt treatment of the disease in order to shorten the disease duration or prolong life is known as

a) Primary prevention b) Secondary prevention

c) Tertiary prevention d) Primordial prevention

52 Type of prevention which modifies the determinants to prevent or postpone new cases of disease is known as

a) Primary prevention b) Secondary prevention

c) Tertiary prevention d) Primordial prevention

53 Which of the followings is not a strategy for control and eradication of disease

a) Quarantine b) Slaughter

c) Doing nothing d) None of the above

54 The routine collection of information on disease, productivity and other characteristic related to them in a population is known as

a) Surveillance b) Monitoring

c) Screening d) Survey

55 A more intensive form of data recording is known as

a) Surveillance b) Monitoring

c) Screening d) Survey

56 Which of the followings detects subclinical and carrier cases by sampling from clinically normal animals

a) Active surveillance b) Passive surveillance

c) Mass screening d) Sentinel surveillance

57 Which of the followings involves examination of clinically affected cases only

a) Active surveillance b) Passive surveillance

c) Mass screening d) Sentinel surveillance

58 Which of the followings involves identification of undiagnosed cases using rapid tests

a) Active surveillance b) Passive surveillance

c) Screening d) Sentinel surveillance

59 Which of the followings is not a part of observational study

a) Cohort study b) Case control study

c) Randomized control trial d) Correlational study

60 Experimental study is associated with

a) Hypothesis formulation b) Hypothesis testing

c) Hypothesis confirmation d) None of the above

61 Analytical study is associated with

a) Hypothesis formulation b) Hypothesis testing

c) Hypothesis confirmation d) None of the above

62 Which of the followings is known as 'cause to effect study'

a) Cohort study b) Case control study

c) Cross sectional study d) Correlational study

63 Which of the followings is known as 'effect to cause study'

a) Cohort study b) Case control study

c) Cross sectional study d) Correlational study

64 Which of the followings is known as 'SNAPSHOT of population study'

a) Cohort study b) Case control study

c) Cross sectional study d) Correlational study

65 Unit of randomized controlled trial is

a) Individual b) Population

c) Patients d) None of the above

66 The ability of a diagnostic test to detect true negatives is known as

a) Sensitivity b) Specificity

c) Positive predictive value d) Positive likelihood ratio

67 The probability that an animal tested positive is actually positive is known as

a) Sensitivity b) Specificity

c) Positive predictive value d) Negative predictive value

68 Positive likelihood ratio of perfect diagnostic test is

a) Zero b) 1

c) -1 d) Infinite

69 In a population of 5000 cattle, 250 cattle were affected with hemorrhagic septicemia out of which 50 animals have died. Find out the mortality and case fatality rate.

a) 5% and 10% b) 1% and 20%

c) 2% and 10% d) 10% and 20%

70 Field epidemiology is also known as

a) Clinical epidemiology b) Shoe leather epidemiology

c) Field trial d) None of the above

Answer Key

1	a	**2**	c	**3**	b	**4**	c	**5**	b	**6**	d	**7**	a	**8**	a	**9**	c	**10**	d
11	a	**12**	b	**13**	d	**14**	c	**15**	c	**16**	b	**17**	a	**18**	d	**19**	a	**20**	b
21	d	**22**	c	**23**	d	**24**	d	**25**	b	**26**	c	**27**	a	**28**	d	**29**	a	**30**	b
31	c	**32**	d	**33**	b	**34**	a	**35**	d	**36**	a	**37**	b	**38**	c	**39**	a	**40**	b
41	d	**42**	a	**43**	d	**44**	c	**45**	d	**46**	b	**47**	a	**48**	b	**49**	d	**50**	c
51	b	**52**	a	**53**	d	**54**	b	**55**	a	**56**	a	**57**	b	**58**	c	**59**	c	**60**	c
61	b	**62**	a	**63**	b	**64**	c	**65**	c	**66**	b	**67**	c	**68**	d	**69**	b	**70**	b

26

Miscellaneous Exercise I

Encircle the right answer from multiple choices

1 Deficiency of which of the following trace minerals leads to parakeratosis of skin in pigs

a) Zinc b) Copper

c) Cobalt d) Iron

2 Milk fever is more common in

a) Indigenous cows b) Holstein cows

c) Jersey cows d) Gir

3 White muscle disease is caused by

a) Excess of selenium b) Deficiency of vitamin C

c) Deficiency of vitamin E d) Excess of Vitamin A

4 The major signs of equine colic

a) Circling, laying down, rolling, and rising frequently

b) Turning the head and looking at the flank or abdomen

c) Kicking at the abdomen, stretching out and standing for long periods

d) All of the above

5 Vaccination failure is more common in FMD because of

a) Antigenic drift of the viral pathogen

b) Poor immune triggering following vaccination

c) Oral route is the recommended for administration

d) Poor antige necity of the vaccine

6 Tachycardia refers to

a) Increase in heart rate and force b) Increase in heart rate only

c) Decrease in heart rate only d) Decrease in heart rate and force

7 Bacterial disease associated with clinical signs referable to meningioence phalitis

a) Leptospirosis b) Listeriosis

c) Anthrax d) Haemorrhagic septicemia

8 Overcrowding of animals predisposes them to diseases. Therefore, the stocking density is required to be collected during history taking. Such information from the owner falls under

a) Physical examination b) Disease history

c) Management history d) Environment history

9 Punched ulcer in abomasums is a pathognomonic post mortem lesion in

a) Babesiosis b) Anaplasmosis

c) Theleriosis d) Cryptococcosis

10 Wound size does not correspond to shape and size of the weapon, the edges of wound are torn and irregular and bleeding may or may not occur and the healing process is very slow in

a) Incised wound b) Contused wound

c) Lacerated wound d) Gunshot wound

11 Koch's blue bodies is seen in lymph node biopsies in

a) Babesiosis b) Anaplasmosis

c) Cryptococcosis d) Theileriosis

12 Use of sharp object is suspected in which of the following wounds

a) Abrasion b) Bruise

c) Laceration d) Incised wounds

13 Urolithiasis is more commonly seen in bullocks and is predisposed by

a) Reduced water intake b) Soil mineral composition

c) Dietary factors d) All of the above

14 Found dead and crepitating sound in muscle are seen in

a) Black Quarters b) Anthrax

c) Lighting stroke d) Haemorrhagic septicemia

15 Rabies should be differentiated from poisoning of

a) Copper b) Lead

c) Arsenic d) Selenium

16 Yellowish discolouration of conjunctiva is seen in

a) Spleenomegally b) Severe renal damage

c) Severe hepatic damage d) Poor blood perfusion to eyes

17 Frequent urination with passage of small amount of urine is seen in

a) Cystitis b) Partial urolithiasis

c) Urethriits d) All of the above

18 Exotoxin is

a) A lipopolysaccharide b) Protein in nature

c) Produced after the death of the organisms d) Not excreted by living cells

19 Leukopenia is mostly seen in

a) Viral diseases b) Acute bacterial diseases

c) Chronic bacterial diseases d) Diseases caused by allergens

20 The white layer between plasma and packed cells in hemogram represents

a) Mature erythrocytes b) Leukocytes

c) Ghost cells d) Only monocytes

21 Aplastic anaemia is manifested by

a) Hypochromic normocytic RBC

b) Hyperchromic normocytic RBC

c) Hypochromic normocytic RBC

d) Normocytic normochromic RBC

22 Abortion in the last trimester of pregnancy in a herd is possibly due to

a) Vibriosis b) Brucellosis

c) Infectious pustular volvovaginitis d) Tuberculosis

23 Peat Scour is commonly seen in

a) Copper deficiency b) Molybdenum deficiency

c) Cobalt deficiency d) Zinc deficiency

24 Piglet anaemia occurs due to

a) Copper deficiency b) Molybdenum deficiency

c) Cobalt deficiency d) Iron deficiency

25 Roaring sound is common in paralysis of

a) Larynx b) Pharynx

c) Tongue d) Face

26 The normal body temperature of a two year old heifer is

a) 100°F b) 101.5°F

c) 102.5°F d) 103°F

27 Intestinal obstruction does not affect

a) Motility of the gastrointestinal tract

b) Mucous production into the intestinal tract

c) Consistency of the faeces

d) None of the above

28 The rational approach in reducing incidence of metabolic diseases in a herd are

a) By regular monitoring of the few metabolic parameters and taking necessary corrective feeding measures

b) Culling of animals prone to the diseases

c) Feeding of protein rich diet

d) All of the above

29 Ultrasonography is a

a) Non-invasive diagnostic technique

b) Semi-invasive diagnostic technique

c) Invasive diagnostic technique

d) Not a diagnostic technique

30 The compensatory mechanism of releasing erythrocytes from the spleen in response to physiological demand is maximum in

a) Cattle b) Pigs

c) Horses d) Sheep

31 Course of the disease refers to the duration from

a) Invasion to establishment of infection

b) Invasion to appearance of the clinical signs

c) Appearance of clinical signs to the ultimate disease outcome

d) Infection to the end of the disease process

32 Epilepsy is a clinical condition characterized by

a) Hyperstheisa

b) Involuntary urination and defecation

c) Unconsciousness about the surrounding for a short period

d) All of the above

33 Sub Acute Ruminal Acidosis (SARA) is a common complication

a) In high yielding animals with rich carbohydrate feeding
b) In cattle fed with high fiber diet
c) Manifested by enteritis and constipation
d) Associated with fall in ruminal pH below 5

34 Lot of mucous on perrectal examination without any faecal material is an indication of

a) Rumenitis b) Intestinal obstruction
c) Hepatic insufficiency d) Abomasal displacement

35 Endoscope can be used in dogs to diagnose ulcerative lesions in the

a) Stomach b) Pylorus
c) Duodenum d) All of the above

36 Vitamin B12 deficiency causes

a) Normocytic anaemia b) Microcytic anaemia
c) Macrocytic anaemia d) All of the above

37 Mean corpuscular haemoglobin (MCV) is a haematological index that reflects

a) The cell size of erythrocytes
b) Hemoglobin content of erythrocytes
c) Anisocytosis
d) None of the above

38 Circling in cattle is seen in following conditions

a) Cadmium poisoning b) Rabies
c) Nervous form of ketosis d) Hyperglycemia

39 Bishoping of animals is punishable under IPC

a) 379 b) 320
c) 420 d) 378

40 In case of ruminal impaction, fluid therapy is recommended along with oral administration of

a) Calcium carbonate b) Sodium silicate
c) Magnesium sulphate d) Potassium iodide

41 Shift to left in blood cells formation indicates

a) More number of mature RBC in circulation
b) More number of immature cells in the circulation
c) Increased in fragility of the cells
d) More number of ghost cells in circulation

42 Metritis-Mastitis-Agalactia (MMA) syndrome is a common problem in

a) Dogs b) Pigs

c) Cows d) Buffaloes

43 Vertigo is a disorder that is referrable to

a) Central nervous system b) Cardiovascular system

c) Respiratory system d) Renal system

44 Cardiac sound can be best asculted on the left side at

a) 4-5th intercostals space b) 5-6th intercostals space

c) 6-7th intercostals space d) 7-8th intercostals space

45 The post-mortem examination is not carried out in suspected cases of anthrax as

a) Spore formation takes place upon exposure to adverse condition

b) The spores survives in soil for a long period

c) The disease has zoonotic significance

d) All of the above

46 Blood loss due to blood sucking parasites like ticks and hook worms is classified under

a) Hemolytic anaemia b) Hemorrhagic anaemia

c) Nutritional anaemia d) Aplastic anaemia

47 False positive results in Intra-dermal tuberculin test refers to those

a) show reaction but are not infected with Microbacterium

b) Infected but does not show reaction

c) Infected and show reaction

d) Do not show reaction and not infected

48 The methylene blue staining of blood smear from a HS patient shows

a) Biopolar staining b) Blue and green staining

c) Spherical organism d) All of the above

49 Cystitis is characterized by

a) Increased frequency of urination

b) Change in urine specific gravity

c) Painful urination

d) All of the above

50 Chorea is

a) Characterized by involuntary, purposeless, spasmodic movements of the entire body or group of muscles

b) Noticed in dogs recovered from canine hepatitis

c) Manifestation referable to autonomic nervous system

d) None of above

51 Rise in the cortisol level at the time of parturition is of

a) Foetal origin
b) Maternal origin
c) Placental origin
d) Both foetal and maternal origin

52 Parasites those lay eggs containing well developed larva are called

a) Oviparous parasites
b) Larviparous parasites
c) Viviparous parasites
d) Ovo-vivi parous parasites

53 Rigor mortis is a

a) Pathological change
b) Post mortem change
c) Antemortem change
d) Death process

54 Immunoglobulin is produced by

a) T cell
b) Plasma cell
c) Cytotoxic cell
d) NK cell

55 The terms like 'epidemic' and 'endemic' were first used by

a) Socrates
b) Fracastoro
c) Hippocrates
d) Robert Koch

56 Number of canine teeth in cattle is

a) One pair
b) Two pairs
c) Three pairs
d) Absent

57 The colour of the plasma depends on

a) Concentration of bilirubin in plasma

b) Species of the animal

c) The quantities stored

d) All of the above

58 The most effective sign to distinguish pyometra from early pregnancy in cow is

a) Presence of cervical seal
b) Double fold membrane
c) Presence of corpus luteum
d) None of the above

59 Follicular mange is caused by

a) Demodex b) Sarcoptes

c) Psoroptes d) All of the above

60 Major teratologic defects arise at the following stage

a) Ovum b) At the time of fertilization

c) Embryo d) Blastocyst formation

61 In MPD, the ligament that is surgically severed is

a) Middle patellar ligament b) Medial patellar ligament

c) Lateral patellar ligament d) Anterior patellar ligament

62 Hypothermia usually develops due to

a) Depletion of glycogen from skeletal muscle

b) Exhaustion of the metabolic process

c) Fall in glycogen content in cardiac muscle

d) All of these

63 The molecular weight of immunoglobulin is the highest in

a) IgM b) IgG

c) IgA d) IgE

64 The chief refracting medium of eye ball is

a) Cornea b) Aquous humour

c) Lens d) Vitreous humour

65 Histidine is converted to histamine by

a) Decarboxylation b) Transamination

c) Hydroxylation d) Phosphorylation

66 The biggest blood cell in mammal is

a) Eosinophil b) Basophil

c) Lymphocyte d) Monocyte

67 The most common cause of seminal vesiculitis is by the organism

a) *Pseudomonas aeruginosa* b) *Brucella abortus*

c) I.B.R. / I.P.V. d) *Corynobacterium pyogenes*

68 Morphologically *Pasteurella multocida* is a

a) Gram –ve bipolar organism b) Gram +ve Cocobacilli

c) Gram –ve bacilli d) Gram +ve Cocci

69 Retained foetal membrane for more than 8-12 hours can have fatal consequences in

a) Bitch b) Mare

c) Sow d) Doe

70 In rabies, inclusion bodies are

a) Intronuclear

b) Intracytoplasmic

c) Both Intra, nuclear and Intracytoplasmic

d) None of the above

71 The most preferred drug for the treatment of Theileriosis is

a) Amitraz b) Diminazene

c) Antrycide prosalt d) Buparvaquone

72 Surra is caused by

a) Trypanosoma *evansi* b) Trypanosoma *vivax*

c) Trypanosoma *equinum* d) All of the above

73 The organism with cork screw like morphology

a) Clostridia b) Chlamydia

c) Leptospira d) Brucella

74 Seasonal anoestrous in sheep is indirectly regulated by

a) Hypothalamus b) Pituitary

c) Pineal gland d) Ovaries

75 Glanders is otherwise known as

a) Equine influenza b) Equine tuberculosis

c) Equine fever d) Farcy

76 During expiration, the intra-pleural pressure

a) Rises b) Decreases

c) Does not change d) None of the above

77 Scarlet fever is caused by

a) *Staphylococcus* species b) *Streptococcus pyogens* gr. A

c) Microfilariae d) *Babesia bigemina*

78 The following condition is noticed in actinomycosis in cattle

a) Dropped jaw b) Bottle jaw

c) Locked jaw d) Lumpy jaw

79 Egg of *paramphistomum* posses

a) Spine b) Operculum

c) Tail d) Flagellum

80 Moniezia *expansa* is a common tape worm of:

a) Cattle b) Dog

c) Poultry d) Horse

81 Avian Leucosis Complex is caused by

a) Herpes virus b) Adeno virus

c) Retro virus d) Irrido virus

82 The primary lymphoid organ of bird is

a) Lymph node b) Spleen

c) Bursa d) Thymus

83 In calcium homeostasis, the minor correction is achieved by hormone

a) Glucagon b) Calcitonin

c) Insulin d) Parathyroid hormone

84 Ketosis in milch cow is attributed to imbalance in input and output related to metabolism of which of the following nutrient

a) Protein b) Minerals

c) Carbohydrates d) Vitamins

85 Snoring disease in cattle is caused by

a) *Schistosoma spindale* b) *Schistosoma nasale*

c) *Schistosoma indicum* d) None of the above

86 PO_2 in the alveolar air is

a) 160 mm Hg b) 105 mm Hg

c) 95 mm Hg d) 45 mm Hg

87 FMD is caused by

a) Adeno virus b) Apthus virus

c) Herpes virus d) Orbi virus

88 Bird flu virus belongs to the family of

a) Paramixoviridae b) Orthomiyxo viridae

c) Retro viridae d) Corona viridae

89 Disease caused by *Fasciola* species as per SNOAPAD can be named as

a) Fascioloses b) Fascioliasis

c) Fasciolosis d) All of the above

90 Usual method of transmission of tularemia is through

a) Infected water b) Infected arthropods

c) Inhalation d) Direct contact

91 *Schistosoma* spp. are commonly called as

a) Blood flukes b) Rumen flukes

c) Liver flukes d) Lung fluke

92 The counter stain used in acid fast staining is

a) Alkaline methylene blue b) Polychrome methylene blue

c) Concentrated Carbol fuschin d) Neutral red

93 Epidemic typhus is caused by

a) *Babesia typhi* b) *Chlamydia pscitassi*

c) *Rickettsia prowazekii* d) *Mycoplasma*

94 Marked swelling of the sciatic nerve in poultry is observed in

a) Lymphoid leucosis b) Ranikhet disease

c) Marek's disease d) Avian encephalomyelitis

95 Red water disease in cattle is caused by

a) *Babesia cobali* b) *Babesia bovis*

c) *Babesia bigemina* d) *Babesia ovis*

96 The longest known cestoda is

a) *Diphilobothrium latum* b) *Taenia solium*

c) *Diphylidium caninum* d) *Moniezia* sps.

97 Pulse rate in cattle is recorded by the palpation of

a) Middle coccygeal artery b) Facial artery

c) Middle sacral artery d) Femoral artery

98 Vaccine used for the control of *Pestes des petites ruminant* (PPR) is

a) Live attenuated b) Inactivated vaccine

c) Oil adjuvant d) Sub-unit vaccine

99 Tuberculin test in cattle herd is performed through

a) Intradermal route b) Subcutaneous route

c) Intramuscular route d) Intraperitoneal route

100 Geographical location where the environment offers favourable conditions for occurrence, maintenance and propagation of a disease is called

a) Niche　　b) Nosoarea

c) Ecology　　d) Nosogenic territory

Answer Key

1	a	**2**	c	**3**	c	**4**	d	**5**	a	**6**	b	**7**	b	**8**	c	**9**	c	**10**	c
11	d	**12**	d	**13**	d	**14**	a	**15**	b	**16**	c	**17**		**18**	b	**19**	a	**20**	b
21	d	**22**	b	**23**	a	**24**	d	**25**	a	**26**	b	**27**	d	**28**	a	**29**	a	**30**	c
31	c	**32**	d	**33**	a	**34**	b	**35**	d	**36**	c	**37**	a	**38**	c	**39**	c	**40**	c
41	b	**42**	b	**43**	a	**44**	a	**45**	d	**46**	b	**47**	a	**48**	a	**49**	d	**50**	a
51	a	**52**	d	**53**	d	**54**	b	**55**	c	**56**	d	**57**	d	**58**	b	**59**	a	**60**	c
61	b	**62**	a	**63**	a	**64**	c	**65**	a	**66**	d	**67**	d	**68**	a	**69**	b	**70**	b
71	d	**72**	a	**73**	c	**74**	c	**75**	d	**76**	a	**77**	b	**78**	d	**79**	b	**80**	a
81	c	**82**	c	**83**	b	**84**	a	**85**	b	**86**	b	**87**	b	**88**	b	**89**	c	**90**	b
91	a	**92**	a	**93**	c	**94**	c	**95**	c	**96**	a	**97**	a	**98**	a	**99**	a	**100**	d

27

Miscellaneous Exercise II

Encircle the right answer from multiple choices

1 Goose stepping gait is observed due to deficiency of

a) Biotin b) Pyrodoxin

c) Pantothenic acid d) Niacian

2 Ranikhet Disease virus is inoculated in developing chicken embryo through

a) Allantoic route b) Amniotic route

c) Yolk sac route d) CAM route

3 The mordant used in Gram's method of staining is

a) Crystal violet b) Diluted Carbol fuchsin

c) Methylene blue d) Gram's iodine

4 Haemolytic anemia is seen in

a) Coccidiosis b) Trypanosomiasis

c) Babesosis d) All of the above

5 In poultry, *Eimeria tenella* causes

a) Caecal coccidiosis b) Intestinal coccidiosis

c) Rectal coccidiosis d) Hepatic coccidiosis

6 Iron deficiency causes

a) Macrocytic hypochromic anaemia

b) Macrocytic normoochromic anaemia

c) Microcytic hypochromic anaemia

d) Microcytic normoochromic anaemia

7 Fever is the combination of

a) Bacteraemia and shock b) Shock and pyrexia

c) Toxaemia and hyperthermia d) Haemolysis and hyperthermia

8 The normal range of ruminal pH in cattle is

a) 6.5-7.5 b) 8.0-8.5

c) 5.5-6.3 d) None of the above

9 Microscopic examination of the skin scrapping is done after digestion of samples with

a) 10% NaCl b) 1% KOH

c) 10% KOH d) 10% HCl

10 Post parturient hemoglobunuria is predisposed by deficiency of

a) Calcium b) Copper

c) Phosphorus d) Zinc

11 Physical examination of recording temperature in large animals is carried out by inserting the thermometer into

a) Oral cavity b) Rectum

c) Vagina d) Either of the above

12 Clinical manifestation of saw-horse posture indicates

a) Lead poisoning b) Tetanus

c) Rabies d) Ruminal acidosis

13 The common post mortem finding in ketosis is

a) Fatty infiltration of liver b) Myelin sheath degeneration

c) Rumen impaction d) Congestion of lungs

14 The type of hypoxia produced in cyanide poisoning

a) Anoxic hypoxia b) Anaemic hypoxia

c) Histotoxic hupoxia d) None of the above

15 Dribbling of urine in a pregnant cow is a common clinical sign in cases of

a) Metritis b) Cystitis

c) Partial urolithiasis d) Urethritis

16 In cases of veterolegal cases, the summon is issued to the accused in

a) Single copy b) Duplicate

c) Triplicate d) Does not matter

17 Scald is seen in cases of

a) Contused wound b) Lacerated wound

c) Burn injury due to dry heat d) Frost bite

18 Anoxia caused due to defective oxygenation of blood in pulmonary circulation is called

a) Anoxic anoxia b) Anaemic anoxia
c) Stagnant anoxia d) Histotoxic anoxia

19 Ruminal atony is observed in

a) Lactic acidosis b) Endotoxemia
c) Abomasal displacement d) Both (a) and (b)

20 Plasma clearance test to examine the liver function is performed using

a) PSB b) BSP
c) Xylitol d) Methylene blue

21 Abnormal frequent passage of urine is known as

a) Oliguria b) Anuria
c) Pollakiuria d) Polyurea

22 Laminitis in cattle is seen as a sequel to

a) Bloat b) Ruminal acidosis
c) TRP d) Vagal indigestion

23 Hyperthermia may be caused due to

a) Iodism b) Dehydration
c) Excessive muscular activity d) All of the above

24 Rupture of pulmonary artery primarily causes

a) Congestive heart failure b) Acute heart failure
c) Peripheral circulatory failure d) All of the above

25 Urticaria occurs due to

a) Allergic reaction b) Photosensitization
c) Iodine deficiency d) Copper deficiency

26 Difficulty in defecation accompanied with straining and tenesmus is observed in

a) Diarrhoea b) Constipation
c) Paralysis of anal spincter d) All of the above

27 The rupture of bladder is more commonly seen in

a) Dogs b) Cattle
c) Goats d) Horses

28 Lack of fluid intake leads to

a) Depression of tissue fluid level

b) Compensatory reduction in fluid output

c) Catabolism of fat, protein and carbohydrate

d) All of the above

29 Ante-mortem wound has

a) No bleeding from the wound

b) Cutting edges not separated

c) Seration of skin cut surfaces even with the use of sharp knife

d) Absence of signs of inflammation

30 Man satisfying his lust through an animal is termed as

a) Bishoping b) Bestiality

c) Tribadism d) Sodomy

31 Vaccination against Marek's disease in poultry is done

a) In day old chick b) At One month

c) At two months d) At 6 months of age

32 Milk fever can be successfully treated with

a) Infusion of antibacterial agents along with calcium salts

b) Intravenous administration of calcium salt

c) High doses of vitamin D

d) Intravenous infusion of magnesium salts

33 The characteristic feature of rabies

a) Roaring sound b) Descending paralysis

c) No control over urine flow d) Chorea

34 Consulting the past clinician who was looking after the patient before advising treatment is a/an/for

a) Legal binding

b) Ethical issue

c) Building relationship

d) Getting clue for future treatment

35 Rabies should be differentiated from poisoning of

a) Molybdenum b) Lead

c) Arsenic d) Selenium

36 Coffee colour urine in babesiosis is due to

a) Internal haemolysis b) Internal haemorrhage

c) Renal damage d) Rupture of bladder

37 Swine influenza is caused by influenza virus of strain

a) H1N1 b) H5N1

c) H9N1 d) H1N5

38 Ascolis test is done for diagnosis of

a) Black Quarters b) Anthrax

c) Haemorrhagic septicemia d) Tuberculosis

39 Which of the following physical examinations is important in diagnosis of ascites in a dog?

a) Palpation b) Ballottement

c) Tactile Percussion d) Succusion

40 The most important aspect of clinical examination in Veterinary Practice is

a) Examination of animal b) Examination of Environment

c) History taking d) Physical examination

41 The major cause of hyperthermia is

a) High environmental temperature b) Bacterial Disease

c) Viral Disease d) All of the above

42 Which of the following examination can be done from a distance

a) Inspection b) Perception

c) Percussion d) Auscultation

43 The initial choice of infusion in case of endotoxemia is

a) Hypertonic solution b) Hypotonic solution

c) Isotonic solution d) Colloidal solution

44 The pH of blood in healthy animal

a) 6.8-7.0 b) 7.1-7.3

c) 7.2-7.4 d) 7.5-7.6

45 Diaphragmatic hernia is most common in which of the following species

a) Cattle b) Buffalo

c) Sheep & Goat d) Horse

46 The common sequel of TRP is

a) Vagus indigestion b) Diaphragmatic hernia

c) Congestive heart failure d) All of the above

47 Ingestion of large amount of undigested carbohydrate food in ruminant leads to

a) Lactic acidosis b) Simple indigestion

c) Vagus indigestion d) None of the above

48 Hay's sulphur test is done to detect

a) Bile Pigment b) Bile salt

c) Ketone body d) Glucose

49 Colour of faeces in obstructive jaundice is

a) Tarry b) Clay

c) Brown d) Yellow

50 Anaemia that occurs due to deficiency of iron is

a) Normocytic normochromic b) Macrocytic hypochromic

c) Microcytic hypochromic d) Microcytic normochromic

51 Arrhythmia is the most common cause of

a) Congestive heart failure b) Acute heart failure

c) Endocarditis d) All of the above

52 ECG picture of 1st degree heart block

a) Prolonged P-R interval b) Prolong P-Q interval

c) Absence of QRS complex d) Peaked T wave

53 Biot's respiration usually observed in

a) Meningitis b) Diabetic ketoacidosis

c) Nephritis d) Cerebral haemorrhage

54 Deep guttural sound originating from vibration of pharyngeal mucosa is called as

a) Snorting b) Stridor

c) Wheezing d) Stretor

55 Which of the following is a bronchodialator for cattle

a) Doxapram b) Pictotoxin

c) Caffeine d) Salbutamol

56 Normal Pulse and Respiration ratio is approximately

a) 2:1 b) 3:1

c) 4:1 d) 5:1

57 Lactation tetany in mare usually occurs due to deficiency of

a) Ca b) Mg

c) P d) Glucose

58 Lactation tetany in cow usually occurs due to deficiency of

a) Ca b) Mg

c) P d) Glucose

59 Oral dosing of zinc oxide in ewes may lead to

a) Hypocalcemia b) Hypomagnesaemia

c) hypophospetemia d) Hypoglycaemia

60 Normal serum level of calcium in healthy cow is

a) 7-9 mg/dl b) 9-11 mg/dl

c) 3-5 mg/dl d) 1.3 -3 mg/dl

61 Ketosis may occur due to nutritional deficiency of

a) Ca b) Mg

c) Co d) Cu

62 Downers cow syndrome is most common in

a) Jersey b) Holstein

c) Non-descriptive desi d) Guernsey

63 Eclampsia in bitch is associated with

a) Hypoglycaemia b) Hypocalcemia

c) Both of the above d) None of the above

64 Parakeratosis occurs due to deficiency of

a) Copper b) Zinc

c) Cobalt d) Sodium

65 The tolerable level of fluoride in a drinking water in animal is

a) 0.5 ppm b) 0.1 ppm

c) 1 ppm d) 5 ppm

66 The co-factor of enzyme Ceruloplasmin oxidase is

a) Co b) Cu

c) Zn d) Se

67 Enzootic muscular dystrophy occurs due to deficiency of

a) Cu b) Co

c) Selenium d) Manganese

68 Colour of mucous membrane in HCN poisoning is

a) Chacolate b) Red

c) Bright red d) Pink

69 Which type of diarrhoea is caused enterotoxic colibacillosis in calf?

a) Osmotic b) Secretory

c) Hypermotility d) Inflammatory

70 The causative agent of black disease is

a) *Clostridium novyi* type B b) *Clostridium chauvoei*

c) *Haemophyleu* species d) *Hemotophysalis* species

71 Post weaning diarrhoea and oedema in pigs is caused by

a) *Salmonella suis* b) *E. coli*

c) Rota virus d) Corona Virus

72 Surra is fatal in which species, if not promptly treated

a) Cattle b) Buffalo

c) Horse d) Camel

73 Three days fever in bovine is caused by

a) Flavi Virus b) Ephemero virus

c) Herpes Virus d) Reo virus

74 Which of the following species shows resistance to FMD?

a) Cattle b) Buffalo

c) Horse d) Elephant

75 Hard pad disease in canine is caused by

a) Adeno virus b) Morbilli virus

c) Parvo virus d) Rhabdo virus

76 The dose rate of buparvaqone (kg body weight) to treat theileriosis in cattle is

a) 1 mg b) 2.5 mg

c) 5 mg d) 10 mg

77 The recommended duration of doxycycline in dog against Ehrlichiosis is

a) One week b) Two weeks

c) Three weeks d) Four weeks

78 Ivermectin is contraindicated in which breed of dog

a) Labrador b) Coolie

c) German Shepherd d) Chihuahua

79 Day old vaccination in chicks is given for protection against which of the following diseases.

a) Pullorum Disease b) Mareks Disease

c) RD d) None of the above

80 Which of the following drugs is contraindicated in demodecosis?

a) Amitraz b) Permethrine

c) Corticosteriod d) Benzyl Peroxide

81 Pulmonary emphysema may lead to

a) Inspiratory dyspnoea b) Expiratory dyspnoea

c) Crackle d) Wheezes

82 Black tongue in dog is due to deficiency of

a) Folic acid b) Vit-A

c) Vit-D3 d) Nicotinic acid

83 California mastitis test detects

a) Change in pH b) Change in leukocyte

c) Both (a) and (b) d) Change in lymphocyte

84 Anal rubbing is a pathognomonic sign of infestation with which of the following parasites

a) *Ancylostoma caninum* b) *Toxocara canis*

c) *Dyphylidium caninum* d) *Dirofilaria immitis*

85 The shape of abdomen in ascities is

a) Apple b) Papple

c) Pear d) Drum

86 Acidic urine usually predisposes to which type of urinary crystal in dog

a) Urate b) Oxalate

c) Struvite d) Cystine

87 Chronic renal failure usually leads to

a) Anuria b) Polyuria

c) Oligouria d) All of the above

88 Which of the following breeds of dog is more prone to urate crystal

a) Labrador b) Spitz

c) Dalmatian d) German Shepherd

89 Bran like deposits on skin is called

a) Urticaria b) Pityriasis

c) Impetigo d) Pachyderma

90 Which of the following conditions is associated with diastolic murmur

a) Mitral insufficiency b) Aortic insufficiency

c) Patent ductus arteriosus d) Pulmonic stenosis

91 Which of the following clinical signs is not associated with heart worm infection in dog

a) Pulmonary Hypertension b) Systemic Hypertension

c) Right Ventricular Hypertrophy d) Pectoral oedema

92 Common cause of chronic blood loss anaemia in young animals is

a) Parasitism b) Copper Deficiency

c) Iron Deficiency d) Immune mediated disease

93 Abomasal impaction leads to

a) Metabolic acidosis b) Metabolic alkalosis

c) Respiratory acidosis d) Respiratory alkalosis

94 White liver disease in sheep occurs due to deficiency of

a) Co b) Cu

c) Mg d) Se

95 Antidote for cyanide poisoning is

a) Sodium thiosulfate b) Sodium Nitrite

c) Charcoal d) Both (a) and (b)

96 Which of the following is a loop diuretics

a) Spiranolactone b) Furesamide

c) Mannitol d) All of the above

97 Presence of undigested blood in the faeces is termed as

a) Haematochezia	b) Odynophagia
c) Hepatodynea	d) None of the above

98 Enzyme deficiency that causes haemolytic anaemia in dog

a) Pyruvate kinase	b) Creatinine Phosphokinase
c) Erythropoietinase	d) Transketolase

99 Ovine ketosis is more common during

a) Early lactation	b) Late pregnancy
c) Early pregnancy	d) Late lactation

100 Presence of cast in urine is an indicative of disease referrable to

a) Kidney	b) Urinary bladder
c) Ureter	d) All of the above

Answer Key

1 c	**2** a	**3** c	**4** c	**5** a	**6** c	**7** c	**8** a	**9** c	**10** c
11 b	**12** b	**13** a	**14** c	**15** c	**16** b	**17** c	**18** a	**19** d	**20** b
21 a	**22** b	**23** d	**24** b	**25** a	**26** b	**27** d	**28** d	**29** d	**30** b
31 a	**32** b	**33** a	**34** b	**35** b	**36** a	**37** a	**38** b	**39** c	**40** c
41 a	**42** a	**43** a	**44** c	**45** b	**46** d	**47** a	**48** b	**49** b	**50** c
51 b	**52** a	**53** a	**54** d	**55** d	**56** c	**57** a	**58** b	**59** a	**60** b
61 c	**62** b	**63** c	**64** b	**65** b	**66** b	**67** c	**68** c	**69** b	**70** a
71 b	**72** c	**73** b	**74** c	**75** b	**76** b	**77** c	**78** b	**79** b	**80** c
81 a	**82** d	**83** c	**84** c	**85** c	**86** b	**87** b	**88** c	**89** b	**90** b
91 b	**92** a	**93** b	**94** a	**95** d	**96** b	**97** a	**98** a	**99** b	**100** a

28

Miscellaneous Exercise III

1 The system that is most susceptible to hypoxia is

a) Respiratory System b) Cardiovascular System

c) Nervous system d) Digestive system

2 Involuntary respiratory movements are influenced by

a) Stretch receptors of lungs

b) Chemoreceptors in carotid body

c) pH of cranial arterial blood supply.

d) All of the above

3 Aplastic anaemia is seen in

a) Copper deficiency b) Cobalt deficiency

c) Radiation injury d) Heat stress

4 Cardiac reserve denotes to

a) Maximum expanding ability of ventricular muscles to accommodate extra volume of blood

b) The amount of blood left over in ventricle after a systolic contraction

c) Maximum stroke volume generating capacity of the heart on demand

d) All of the above

5 Curled toe paralysis in poultry is caused by deficiency of

a) Riboflavin b) Biotin

c) Thiamine d) Pantothenic acid

6 Which of following animals are more succeptibile to haemorrhagic septicemia

a) Cattle b) Buffalo

c) Sheep d) Goat

7 Which of the followings is a common finding in FMD in young calves leading to the death of animal

a) Pericarditis b) Myocarditis

c) Endocarditis d) Pericardial temponade

8 The circling movement in cattle is seen in

a) Babesiosis b) Lactacidemia

c) Listeriosis d) All of the above

9 The nasal schistosomiasis in bovine can be treated with

a) Lithium antimony tartarate b) Levamisol

c) Oxyclosanide d) None of the above

10 The trypanosomiasis in camel is known as

a) Tribursa b) Surra

c) Bibarsa d) Circling disease

11 Pabble shaped abdomen is seen in

a) Ruminal Acidosis b) Alkaline indigestion

c) Vagus indigestion d) Ruminal tympany

12 The clinical signs of dyspnoea is

a) Open mouth breathing b) Protrusion of tongue

c) Increased rate and depth of respiration d) All of the above

13 The causative microorganism is invariably found in the blood stream during

a) Toxemia b) Septicemia

c) Hyperthermia d) All of the above

14 The sternal recumbancy in a newly calved cow is seen in

a) Milk fever 3rd stage b) Milk fever 2nd stage

c) Diaphragmatic hernia d) Ketosis

15 Jaundice due to complete extrahepatic biliary obstruction is associated with

a) Yellowish discolouration of faeces

b) Marked rise in serum level of direct bilirubin

c) Normal colour of the urine

d) Presence of urobilinogen in urine

16 Case fatality rate takes into account

a) No. of animals affected b) No. of affected animals died

c) No of animals exposed to risk d) Both (a) and (b)

17 Difficulty in defecation accompanied with straining and tenesmus is observed in

a) Copper deficiency b) Lead poisoning

c) Rectal paralysis d) All of the above

18 Rectal examination of the cattle may indicate the disease conditions such as

a) Paratuberculosis b) Tuberculosis

c) Colibacillosis d) Salmonellosis

19 Nutritional hemoglobinuria is commonly predisposed by deficiency of

a) Calcium b) Phosphorus

c) Magnesium d) Sodium

20 The antidote used in nitrate and nitrite poisoning is

a) Sodium thiosulfate b) BAL

c) Methylene blue d) Calcium disodium EDTA

21 Which one of the followings is used parenterally as an ecto- and endo-parasital drugs?

a) Albendazole b) Praziquantel

c) Ivermectin d) None of the above

22 Ping sound on percussion over the right abdomen indicates

a) Ruminal acidosis b) Abomasal displacement

c) Vagus indigestion d) Traumatic reticuloperitonitis

23 The dose rate of praziquantel per kg body weight against tape worm infection in bovine is

a) 10 mg b) 5 mg

c) 15 mg d) 20 mg

24 The drug of choice against saprophytic bacteria coming under Clostridial species is

a) Penicillin b) Gentamycine

c) Clavunulic acid d) Tetracyclin

25 The drug of choice against fasciolosis

a) Triquin b) Triclabendazole

c) Levamisole d) Thiacetarsamide

26 ________ infiltration of liver is a common post mortem finding in ketosis

a) Leukocytic b) Neutrophil

c) Eiosonophil d) Fatty

27 Fever is the combination of _________ and

a) Toxaemia and hypothermia b) Toxaemia and hyperthermia

c) Bacteremia and hypothermia d) Bacteremia and hyperthermia

28 Hypoxia caused due to defective oxygenation of blood in pulmonary circulation is

a) Anoxic anoxia b) Anaemic anoxia

c) Stagnant anoxia d) Histotoxic anoxia

29 The sounds of peristalsis is normally heard in cattle during auscultation in the lungs areas on the left side, and those sounds are due to movement of

a) Reticulum b) Lungs

c) Abomasum d) Colon

30 Respiratory failure result into

a) Metabolic acidosis b) Metabolic alkalosis

c) Dehydration d) None of the above

31 In geriatric cats, polydispsia and polyuria are common signs of

a) Hyperthyroidism b) Renal failure

c) Diabetes mellitus d) All of the above

32 Which of the following species has the highest faecal output

a) Horse b) Cattle

c) Sheep and goats d) Pigs

33 Manifestation of pica is seen due to deficiency of

a) Phosphorus b) Calcium

c) Molybdenum d) Zinc

34 The sound emitted by an organ containing air (not under pressure) upon percussion is called

a) Typmpanic b) Resonant

c) Dull d) Loud

35 The distinct systolic and diastolic thumps of the heart sounds are replaced by thrill in

a) Valvular insufficiency b) Valvular stenosis

c) Congential septal defects d) All of the above

36 Fluid thrill is perceived in ascites by

a) Auscultation b) Indirect palpation

c) Tactile percussion d) Direct palpation

37 The time required for digestion of the thread during cellulose digestion test of rumen liquor from a healthy cow is

a) 10 hrs b) 20 hrs

c) 30 hrs d) 40 hrs

38 Forthy tympany in ruminants occurs due to feeding on

a) Lucern b) Bajra grains

c) Maize grain d) Jowar grains

39 A clinically effective bone marrow stimulant is

a) Iron salt b) Cyanocobalamine

c) DL-Batyl alcohol d) Acyclovir

40 The agent that counteracts the effects (pharmacological/ physiological) of a poison or removes it from the body is known as

a) Aphasia b) Antidote

c) Aperients d) Cathartic

41 Which of the following is liver specific enzyme in cattle

a) SGPT (ALT) b) SGOT (AST)

c) Sorbitol dehydrogenase d) Alkaline phosphatase

42 Which of the followings is not linked to kidney function test

a) PSP Clearance test b) Creatinine clearance test

c) BSP clearance test d) Blood Urea Nitrogen

43 Clinically, icterus in ruminants is most frequently associated with

a) Haemolytic crisis b) Liver damage

c) Biliary Stasis d) All of the above

44 The incidence of milk fever depends on

a) Genetic and management factors

b) Feeding regimen just prior toparturition

c) Breed of the cow
d) All of the above

45 Sampling should be done from following group of animals for the Compton Metabolic profile test

a) Dry cows
b) Medium yielding lactating cows
c) High yielding lactating cows
d) All of the above

46 Metabolic diseases in sheep has greatest significance in

a) Lactating ewes
b) Female sheep during dry period
c) Pregnant ewes
d) Adult sheep

47 Sound waves from transducer of ultrasound are produced by

a) Piezoelectric crystals
b) Electronic circuit
c) Coupling medium
d) None of the above

48 The principle behind ultrasound scanning with the use of sound waves is

a) Reflection
b) Absorption
c) Scattering
d) Total internal reflection

49 Maximum permissible limits of NVLs reactors in a herd during tuberculin testing by single intra-dermal test is

a) 5%
b) 7%
c) 10%
d) 12%

50 CSF protein is qualitatively detected by

a) Heller's test
b) Gemlin test
c) Sulkowitch test
d) Pandey's test

51 The common complication in canine distemper dogs that refers to disturbance in nervous system

a) Encephalitis
b) Chorea
c) Tetany
d) Hyperesthesia

52 Carbohydrate engorgement in ruminants leads to decline in blood pH due to increase in the blood concentration of

a) Volatile fatty acid
b) Carbonic acid
c) Acetic acid
d) Lactic acid

53 The failure of the right side of the heart shows engorgement of

a) Pulmonary vein
b) Jugular vein
c) Carotid artery
d) None of the above

54 The silhoute of the abdomen in vagus indigestion when seen from the back the animal is

a) Papple shaped b) Apple shaped

c) Drum shaped d) Pear shaped

55 Over feeding proteinous diet or urea in ruminants results in

a) Simple indigestion b) Acid indigestion

c) Alkaline indigestion d) None of the above

56 Obstruction of the esophagus associated with failure in eructation in ruminants results in

a) Primary ruminal tympany b) Secondary ruminal tympany

c) Forthy bloat d) None of the above

57 Collapse of the alveoli due to failure of inflation is known as

a) Atalactasis b) Pneumothorax

c) Hemoptysis d) Dysponea

58 The metabolites produced from chlorophyll present in the green leaves, responsible for photosensitization in bullock is

a) Chlorophyll b b) Erythritol

c) Phylloerythrin d) Calcitonin

59 Dry matter content of hay is

a) 60-70% b) 50-60%

c) 85-90% d) 30-50%

60 The anti-nutritional factor, Gossypol, is present in

a) Ground nut cake b) Linseed meal

c) Cotton seed meal d) Mustard cake

61 Calcium homeostasis in lactating cow is maintained by

a) Parathyroid hormone b) Calcitonin

c) Vitamin-D d) All of the above

62 Probiotic refers to

a) Chemicals b) Same as prebiotic

c) Fat solvent d) Live microbial feed supplement

63 Paddy straw is rich in

a) Oxalic acid b) Calcium

c) Digestible crude protein d) Crude protein

64 The cell wall of gram positive bacteria is composed primarily of

a) Lipid b) Glycerol

c) Polysaccharide d) Peptidoglycan

65 Diamond shaped skin lesions in pigs is characteristic of

a) Black quarter b) Erysipelas

c) Hog cholera d) Swine fever

66 Which of the following is/are correct inr Ranikhet Disease (RD) in poultry

a) Velogenic strain causes encephalic form of the disease

b) Virus belongs to picorna viridae family

c) Haemorrhages in proventriculus noticed during post mortem examination

d) None of the above

67 Inward curling of toes in chicks is caused due to the deficiency of

a) Thiamine b) Riboflavin

c) Biotin d) Cyanocobalamine

68 Parasites with two or more hosts are

a) Hyperparasite b) Heterxenous

c) Monoxenous d) Stenoxenous

69 The host which transfers the infective agent without any development in it

a) Paratenic host b) Transport host

c) Intermediate host d) Reservoir host

70 The association between two different species in which both parasite and host benefits but it is not obligatory, then it is called as

a) Symbiosis b) Parasitism

c) Mutualisim d) Commensalism

71 The mechanical vector for *Trypanosoma evansi* is

a) Culex spp b) *Amblyloma veriegatum*

c) *Rhiphicephalus appendiculatus* d) Tabanus spp

72 Scaly leg in poultry is caused by

a) *Demodex canis* b) *Sarcoptes scabiei*

c) *Notoedres cati* d) *Cnemidocoptes mutans*

73 Benign bovine theleriosis is caused by

a) *Theleria annulata* b) *Theleria parva*

c) *Theleria mutans* d) *Theleria orientalis*

74 Metronidazole is the drug of choice for

a) Coccidiosis b) Entamoebosis

c) Bovine trypanosomosis d) Leshmaniosis

75 What is the most likely cause of death in organophosphate poisoning

a) Gastrointestinal bleeding b) Hypertension

c) Respiratory failure d) Congestive heart failure

76 HCl in the stomach is secreted by

a) Paneth cells b) Goblet cells

c) Parietal cells d) Chief cells

77 Carbohydrate used for the study of glomerular filtration rate (GFR) is

a) Glucose b) Pectin

c) Inulin d) Agar

78 Leukopenia is mostly seen in

a) Bacterial diseases b) Viral diseases

c) Chronic bacterial diseases d) Protozoal diseases

79 Normocytic normochromic anaemia is associated with

a) Haemolytic anaemia

b) Hemorrhagic anaemia

c) Aplastic anaemia due to X ray irradiation

d) Heavy hook work infestation

80 Gid is caused by

a) Adult parasite b) Intermediate stage of parasite

c) Oocyst of the parasite d) Nematode parasite in definite host

81 The wooden tongue in cattle is caused by

a) *Actinobacillus lignieresii* b) *Actinomycosis bovis*

c) *Clostridium tetani* d) *Clostridium botulinum*

82 Stormont test is used to detect which of the following diseases

a) Tuberculosis b) Paratuberculosis

c) Anthrax d) Brucellosis

83 Summer mastitis in cow is caused by

a) *Escherichia coli* b) *Streptococcus agalactiae*

c) *Corynobacterium pyogen* d) *Staphylococcus pyogens*

84 Black Quarter in calves is caused by

a) *Clostridium Perfrigens* b) *Clostridium septicum*

c) *Clostridium botulinum* d) *Clostridium Chauvei*

85 The ideal fluid for the treatment of lactacidemia is

a) 5% Dextrose Saline b) 1.3% Sodium bicarbonate

c) 10% Dextrose Saline d) Normal Saline solution

86 Verminous pneumonia in calves is caused by

a) Ascariasis b) *Pasturella multocida*

c) *Pasturella haemolyticum* d) *Mycobacterium tuberculosis*

87 Bestiality is punishable under section

a) IPC 377 b) IPC 420

c) IPC 379 d) IPC 129

88 *Eimeria tenella* in poultry causes

a) Hepatic coccidiosis b) Renal coccidiosis

c) Caecal coccidiosis. d) intestinal coccidiosis.

89 Rothera's test of urine samples from bovine confirms

a) Milk fever b) Ketosis

c) Hypomagnesemia tetany d) Lactation tetany

90 Potato soup like uterine discharge in bovines occurs ininfection with

a) *Brucella abortus* b) *Trichomonas foetuses*

c) *Escherichia coli* d) *Corynobacterium pyogen*

91 Bleeding of all natural orifices without clotting leading to death is seen in

a) Brucellosis b) Haemorrhagic septicemia

c) *Clostridium haemolyticum* d) Anthrax

92 The circling movement in cattle is seen in

a) Babesiosis b) Lactacidemia

c) Listeriosis d) Leptospirosis

93 The drug of choice for treatment of *Trichomonas fetus* is

a) Sulphonamide b) Lansoprazole

c) Metronidazole d) Penicillin

94 The nasal schistosomiasis in bovine can be treated with
   a) Lithium antimony tartarate b) Levamisole
   c) Oxyclosanide with Levamisol d) Praziquintal

95 Bottle jaw condition in cattle is seen in
   a) Black Quarter b) Fascioliasis
   c) Cestodiosis d) Amphistomiasis

96 The causative microorganism is invariably found in the blood stream during
   a) Toxemia b) Septicemia
   c) Hyperthermia d) Hypothermia

97 Psittacosis in birds is caused by
   a) *Chlamydia psittaci* b) *E. coli*
   c) *Salmonella psittasi* d) *E. psittasi*

98 The trypanosomiasis in camel is known as
   a) Tribursa b) Circling diseases
   c) Bibarsa d) Surra

99 Drum sound on left paralumbar fossa is produced in
   a) Ruminal Acidosis b) Alkaline indigestion
   c) Vagus indigestion d) Ruminal tympany

100 The lateral recumbency in a newly calved cow seen in
   a) Milk fever 3rd stage b) Milk fever 2nd stage
   c) Diaphragmatic hernia d) Ketosis

Answer Key

1	c	**2**	d	**3**	c	**4**	d	**5**	a	**6**	b	**7**	b	**8**	c	**9**	a	**10**	a
11	c	**12**	d	**13**	b	**14**	b	**15**	b	**16**	d	**17**	c	**18**	a	**19**	b	**20**	a
21	c	**22**	b	**23**	b	**24**	a	**25**	b	**26**	d	**27**	b	**28**	a	**29**	a	**30**	a
31	d	**32**	b	**33**	a	**34**	b	**35**	d	**36**	c	**37**	c	**38**	a	**39**	c	**40**	b
41	c	**42**	c	**43**	a	**44**	d	**45**	d	**46**	c	**47**	a	**48**	a	**49**	c	**50**	d
51	b	**52**	d	**53**	b	**54**	a	**55**	c	**56**	b	**57**	a	**58**	c	**59**	c	**60**	c
61	d	**62**	d	**63**	a	**64**	d	**65**	b	**66**	c	**67**	b	**68**	c	**69**	b	**70**	a
71	d	**72**	d	**73**	c	**74**	b	**75**	c	**76**	c	**77**	c	**78**	b	**79**	c	**80**	b
81	a	**82**	a	**83**	c	**84**	d	**85**	a	**86**	a	**87**	a	**88**	c	**89**	b	**90**	b
91	d	**92**	c	**93**	c	**94**	a	**95**	d	**96**	b	**97**	a	**98**	a	**99**	d	**100**	c

29

Miscellaneous Exercise IV

1 The focal point of any disease investigation in animal is making of

a) Treatment b) Diagnosis

c) Management d) Prognosis

2 Forecasting of a disease outcome is termed as

a) Diagnosis b) History taking

c) Prognosis d) Investigation

3 Anaemia that occurs due to failure of regeneration of erythrocytes in the bone marrow

a) Haemolytic b) Haemorrhagic

c) Aplastic d) Iron deficiency anaemia

4 The bacterial that play important role in producing ruminal acidosis following ingestion of highly digestible carbohydrate is

a) *Streptococcus bovis* b) *Lactobacillus ruminaticum*

c) Methanogenic bacteria d) *Staphylococcus bovis*

5 Hyperthermia may be seen following feeding of

a) Strychnine b) Eucalyptus

c) Cyanogenic plant d) Leguminous fodder

6 Traumatic reticulo-peritonitis is characterized by

a) Neutrophillia b) Shift of right

c) Leukopenia d) Neutopenia

7 The superficial lymh node (prescapular) that is palpated for its enlargement for diagnosis of which of the following diseases

a) Babesiosis b) Anthrax

c) Anaplasmosis d) Theileriois

8 Impaired metabolism of (A) carbohydrate/ (B) lipid/ (C) mineralscauses ketosis in ruminants

a) Only A b) Only C

c) Both A and B d) Both A and C

9 Release of which of the following chemical in ruminants into environment is responsible for green house effects

a) Propionic acid b) Methane

c) Acteto acetic acid d) Ammonia

10 Secondary copper deficiency occurs due to

a) Lowered copper content in soil

b) Excess of molybdenum in plants/ fodder

c) Reduced intake of protein rich diet

d) Lowered level of sulfate in the soil

11 The common carrier of leptospirosis is

a) Rodents b) Fishes

c) Bats d) Fomites

12 Corrugation of the intenstine is seen in

a) Strangles b) Paratuberculosis

c) Ephemeral fever d) IBR

13 Hot, painful, emphysematous swelling around the neck region with high rise in body temperature is the common findings in

a) HS b) BQ

c) Braxy d) TB

14 Vaccination confers

a) Innate immunity b) Active immunity

c) Only humoral immunity d) Passive immunity

15 The earliest noticeable clinical signs in tetanus is

a) Saw horse posture b) Prolapse of third eye lid

c) Opisthotonos d) Tetany of hind legs

16 The best method for the control of summer mastitis is

a) Teat dipping b) Dry cow therapy

c) Hygiene d) Culling of mastitic animals

17 California mastitis test detects

a) Change in leukocyte b) Change in pH

c) Change in erythrocyte d) Change in leucocytes and pH

18 The predisposing factor for Black disease in sheep is

a) Clostridium novi b) Clostridium septicum

c) Fasciola hepatica d) Amphistome

19 Silage feeding is associated with

a) Leptospirosis b) Listeriosis

c) Salmonella d) Collibacillous

20 Hygroma of knee joint in calf is an important clinical feature of the disease

a) Strangle b) Tuberculosis

c) Brucellosis d) Leptospirosis

21 Blood in milk during later part of milking arouse suspicion for

a) Listeriosis b) Tetanus

c) Botulism d) Tuberculosis

22 Babesiosis

a) Is a tick borne disease

b) Indigenous cattle are equally susceptible as crossbred

c) Piroplasma are seen only inside the immature RBC

d) Berenil is not effective against babesiosis

23 The comparative tuberculin testing is carried out to

a) Identify anergic cases

b) Distinguish between bovine and avian tuberculosis

c) Distinguish between tuberculosis and Johne's disease

d) None of the above

24 The infective stage of Babesia, injected by ticks is

a) Sporozoits b) Trophozoits

c) Sporocyst d) Piroplasm

25 Which is the most important toxin in *Clostridium perfringens* type-D enterotoxemia?

a) Alfa - toxin b) Beta - toxin

c) Epsilon - toxin d) Gama - toxin

26 Abortion, still birth and metritis is associated with which of the following diseases

a) Brucellosis b) Listeriosis

c) Leptospirosis d) Tuberculosis

27 Chorea in dogs is a common squeal to

a) Infectious canine hepatitis b) Rabies

c) Canine distemper d) Leptospirosis

28 FMD virus belongs to family

a) Reoviridae b) Retroviridae

c) Picornaviridae d) Lentiviridae

29 The common disease of sheep and goat resembling rinderpest in cattle

a) Petis des petites ruminants b) Sheep pox

c) Scrapie d) Louping ill

30 One of the common findings in viral diseases such as Infectious pustular vulvo- vaginitis, mucosal disease and blue tongue

a) Laminitis b) Abortion

c) Diarrhoea d) Myocarditis

31 Pin-worm of horses that causes anal pruritus

a) *Oxyuris equi* b) *Taenia hydatigena*

c) *Haemobartonela equi* d) *Musca domestica*

32 Adult *Fasciola hepatica* is found in

a) Rumen b) Liver

c) Abomasum d) Reticulum

33 Catarrhal stomatitis, rhinitis, enteritis and lameness are characteristic symptoms of which of the following diseases in sheep

a) Petis des petites ruminants b) Sheep pox

c) Blue tongue d) Louping ill

34 Tiger heart and high mortality rate in FMD are seen in

a) Young calves b) Adult cattle

c) Pigs d) Sheep and goats

35 Swine influenza caused by Influenza virus type A belongs to strain

a) H1N1 b) H5N1

c) H5N5 d) H1N5

36 The infective stage in fascioliosis is

a) Eggs b) Sporocyst

c) Cercaria d) Metacercaria

37 Which of the following statements is true about Foot and mouth disease?

a) Affects cloven footed animals only

b) Also affects carnivores

c) Mortality more than 80%

d) Morbidity is around 20%

38 Fascioliasis may predispose to

a) BQ b) Bacillary haemoglobinuria

c) Anthrax d) HS

39 In coeneurosis, the cyst exert pressure on

a) Brain b) Liver

c) Spleen d) Kidney

40 Which of the following statements is correct about Trichomoniasis?

a) Transmitted by coitus

b) Transmitted by blood transfusion

c) It is a non-contagious disease

d) It is a bacterial disease associated with abortion

41 Bovine Virus Diarrhoea is caused by

a) Picorna virus b) Adeno virus

c) Pesti virus d) Retro virus

42 Hyperkeratosis of nose and footpad is a notable feature of

a) Equine distemper b) Canine distemper

c) Equine influenza d) Swine fever

43 Schistosomosis is characterized by clinical signs referable to

a) Nervous system b) Gastrointestinal system

c) Respiratory system d) Urinary system

44 Trypanosoma is

a) Extra erythrocytic protozoa b) Intraerythrocytic protozoa

c) Intra monocytic protozoa d) Intra eisonophil protozoa

45 Which of the following diseases is a sexually transmitted bacterial disease that can cause uveitis, abortion, and orchitis in dog?

a) Leptospirosis b) Listeriosis

c) Brucellosis d) Pasteurellosis

46 Rabies is caused by

a) Paramyxovirus b) Lyssa virus

c) Herpes virus d) Adeno virus

47 Infectious canine hepatitis is caused by

a) Paramyxovirus b) Morbili virus

c) Herpes virus d) Adeno virus

48 The most common cause of death in older cats

a) Chronic kidney failure b) Hepatic failure

c) Cardiac failure d) Respiratory failure

49 Bad breath and bleeding gums; pawing at the mouth; drooling and loss of appetite in cat is seen in

a) Periodontal disease b) Pancreatitis

c) Hypoglycemia d) Hyper thyrodism

50 Oestrus period in dogs lasts for

a) 3-4 days b) 5-7 days

c) 9-10 days d) 15-20 days

51 Vaccination of dogs starts at the age of

a) 6-8 weeks b) 9-11 weeks

c) 16-18 weeks d) 20-22 weeks

52 Exposure to oxidants can denature haemoglobin reslting in

a) Heinz bodies in erythrocytes b) Anisocytosis

c) Megaloblastic erythrocytes d) Microcytic erythrocytes

53 Severe blood loss is a causes of

a) cardiogenic shock b) Hypovolemic shock

c) Septic shock d) Hemolytic shock

54 Which of the following species are more sensitive to Heinz bodies

a) Dog b) Cats

c) Cattle d) Rabbits

55 The Normal Surface antigen of RBC is altered in which of following diseases

a) Listeriosis b) Ehrlichiosis

c) Trypanosomiasis d) Babesiosis

56 The site of erythropoietin production in the kidney is located in

a) Interstitial renal cells
b) Juxta glomerular aparatus
c) Bowman's capsule
d) Distal convoluted tubules

57 The rise in viscosity in polycythemia becomes more pronounced in dogs when the PCV is

a) 20-30%
b) 30-40%
c) 40-50%
d) 50-60%

58 The prognosis for primary polycythemia is

a) Favourable
b) Poor
c) Guarded
d) Good

59 Microcytic hypochromic anaemia is seen in deficiency of

a) Mo
b) Co
c) Fe
d) Mn

60 Cavitation of bone marrow in case of myelophthistic anemia can be detected by

a) ECG
b) Ultrasonography
c) Radiography
d) Differential counting

61 Blood matching in farm animals for blood transfusion is a difficult proposition for which of following reasons

a) Large number of red cell antigens
b) Collection of blood from large animals is time consuming
c) Highly expensive
d) Almost negligible allergic reaction

62 Megaloblastic anemia is encountered in

a) Thiamine deficiency
b) Riboflavin deficiency
c) Vit-B12 deficiency
d) Vit-K deficiency

63 Acute hypovolemic heart failure occurs when the blood loss exceeds

a) 20%
b) 35%
c) 45%
d) 50%

64 Bradykinin released during shock causes pain, vasodilatation & oedema and also stimulates production of

a) Prostaglandin
b) Prostacyclin
c) Erythrocytin
d) Erythropoetin

65 Which of the followings is the principal hormone that regulates RBC production

a) Prostacyclin b) Erythropoietin

c) Prostaglandin d) Erythrocytin

66 The indicator of regenerative anaemia in the blood smear examination is

a) Leukocytosis b) Leukopenia

c) Microcytic RBC d) Reticulocytosis

67 The first blood cell formation in prenatal period is expressed in

a) Bone marrow b) Liver

c) Spleen d) Thymus

68 Polycythemia increases blood

a) Viscosity b) Fluidity

c) Circulation d) Clotting

69 The type of anaemia produced in severe blood sucking parasitism is

a) Haemorrhagic anaemia b) Haemolytic anaemia

c) Aplastic anaemia d) Non-regenerative anaemia

70 Immune mediated hemolytic anaemia shows increased

a) Erythroytic agglutination b) Positive antiglobulin test

c) Both (a) and (b) d) Bleeding time

71 Increased activity of AST is indicative of muscular damage

a) Liver disorders b) Renal disorders

c) Pancreatic insufficiency d) Osteoporosis

72 Bacterial infection of central nervous system is associated with

a) Decreased concentration of protein in CSF

b) Pleocytosis

c) Negative Pandey's test

d) Positive Rothera test

73 Pole test is used for diagnosis of cases of

a) Vagus indigestion b) Traumatic reticuloperitonitis

c) Ruminal acidosis d) Left side abomasal displacement

74 The ST segment in ECG represents the early phase of

a) Atrial contraction b) Ventricular relaxation

c) Atrial relaxation d) Ventricular depolarization

75 Pancreatitis in dogs is associated with increased serum level of

a) Carboxypeptidase A (CPA) b) Creatinine phosphokinase
c) Lactose dehydrogenase d) Aspartate amino transferase

76 Increased CPK level is a good indicator of

a) Renal damage b) Muscular damage
c) Hepatic damage d) Bone dystrophy

77 PSP clearance test is used to detect the

a) Tubular capacity of kidney b) Liver disorder
c) Capacity of the urinary bladder d) Pancreatic disfunction

78 Anergic animals are those with

a) Visible lesions of tuberculosis but do not react to a cutaneous delayed hypersensitivity test
b) Visible lesions of tuberculosis and react to a cutaneous delayed hyper sensitivity test
c) No visible lesion and do not react to a cutaneous delayed hyper sensitivity test
d) No visible lesion but react to a cutaneous delayed hypersensitivity test

79 Vallee's and Sigurdsson vaccine are used to control

a) Anthrax b) Johne's disease
c) Tuberculosis d) CBPP

80 Which of the following is liver specific enzyme in cattle

a) SGPT (ALT) b) SGOT (AST)
c) Sorbitol dehydrogenase d) Alkaline phosphatise

81 Which of the following is not linked to kidney function

a) PSP Clearance test b) Creatinine clearance test
c) BSP clearance test d) Blood Urea Nitrogen

82 Steatorrhoea is a manifestation in dysfunction of

a) Spleen b) Kidney
c) Heart d) Liver

83 The most appropriate diagnostic equipment to detect cardiac arrhythmia in dog is

a) ECG b) EEG
c) Echocardiography d) Laparoscope

84 Sound waves from transducer of ultrasound are produced by

a) Piezoelectric crystals b) Electronic circuit

c) Coupling medium d) None of the above

85 The principle of ultrasound scanning with the use of sound waves is

a) Reflection b) Absorption

c) Scattering d) Total internal reflection

86 Maximum permissible limits of NVLs reactors in a herd for tuberculin testing by single intra-dermal test is

a) 5% b) 7%

c) 10% d) 12%

87 Stormont test is used for screening of which of the following disease

a) Johnes disease b) Tuberculosis

c) CCPP d) Brucellosis

88 CSF protein is qualitatively detected by

a) Heller's test b) Gmelin test

c) Pandey's test d) Sulkowitch test

89 Scintigraphy uses radiopharmaceuticals to produce

a) One dimensional image b) Two dimensional image

c) Three dimensional image d) Multi dimensional image

90 T wave in ECG indicates ventricular

a) Depolarization b) Repolarization

c) Relaxation d) Contraction

91 The common site for collection of CSF is.

a) cistern magna b) Thoraco-lumbar junction

c) Sacro-coccygeal junction d) T3 and T4 joint

92 The Van-den Bergh reaction is used to measure the level of

a) Bile salts b) Billirubin

c) Creatinine d) Serum potassium

93 CSF pressure can be determined by the use of a

a) Manometer b) Stethoscope

c) Barometer d) Thermometer

94 Slow and painful urination is termed as

a) Stranguria b) Oliguria

c) Polyurea d) Dribbling of urine

95 What is the colour of faeces in cases of extra-hepatic bile duct obstruction?

a) Yellow b) Clay

c) Green d) White

96 The normal pH of rumen fluid is

a) 6.2-7.2 b) 7.0-7.8

c) 5.5-6.5 d) 2.0-3.0

97 The appearance of only QRS complex, baseline undulation without P wave in ECG indicates

a) Atrial fibrillation b) Ventricular fibrillation

c) Stenosis of aortic valve d) Stenosis of semilunar valve

98 Which of the following enzyme activity indicates organophosphate toxicity?

a) Beta lactamase b) Lactose dehydrogenase

c) Cholinesterase d) Gamma glutamyl transpeptidase

99 Computed tomography uses which of the followings for taking cross sectional images

a) X-rays b) Gamma rays

c) Ultra sound d) Electronic wavea

100 Apelt's test requires

a) Ammonium sulfate b) Magnesium sulfate

c) Sodium bicarbonate d) Sodium hydroxide

Answer Key

1	b	**2**	c	**3**	a	**4**	a	**5**	a	**6**	a	**7**	d	**8**	c	**9**	b	**10**	b
11	a	**12**	b	**13**	a	**14**	b	**15**	b	**16**	b	**17**	d	**18**	c	**19**	b	**20**	c
21	d	**22**	a	**23**	c	**24**	a	**25**	c	**26**	a	**27**	c	**28**	c	**29**	a	**30**	b
31	a	**32**	b	**33**	c	**34**	a	**35**	b	**36**	d	**37**	a	**38**	b	**39**	b	**40**	a
41	c	**42**	b	**43**	c	**44**	a	**45**	c	**46**	b	**47**	d	**48**	a	**49**	a	**50**	b
51	a	**52**	a	**53**	b	**54**	b	**55**	b	**56**	a	**57**	d	**58**	c	**59**	c	**60**	c
61	a	**62**	b	**63**	a	**64**	b	**65**	b	**66**	d	**67**	b	**68**	a	**69**	a	**70**	c
71	a	**72**	b	**73**	b	**74**	b	**75**	a	**76**	b	**77**	a	**78**	a	**79**	c	**80**	c
81	c	**82**	d	**83**	a	**84**	a	**85**	a	**86**	c	**87**	b	**88**	c	**89**	c	**90**	b
91	a	**92**	b	**93**	a	**94**	a	**95**	b	**96**	c	**97**	a	**98**	c	**99**	a	**100**	a

30

Miscellaneous Exercise V

1 Hypoxia caused due to defective oxygenation of blood in pulmonary circulation

a) Anoxic anoxia b) Anaemic anoxia

c) Stagnant anoxia d) Histotoxic anoxia

2 Acid indigestion in cattle can be treated with

a) Vinegar b) Magnesium sulphate

c) Mineral oil d) Sodium bicarbonate

3 Rapid with shallow breathing is termed as

a) Polypnoea b) Tachypnoea

c) Hyperpnoea d) Dyspnoea

4 Difficulty in defecation accompanied with straining and tenesmus is usually observed in

a) Copper deficiency b) Lead poisoning

c) Rectal paralysis d) All of the above

5 Rectal examination of the cattle may indicate the disease conditions such as

a) Paratuberculosis b) Tuberculosis

c) Colibacillosis d) Salmonellosis

6 Laryngitis is a sequale to

a) Acidosis b) Bloat

c) TRP d) Vagal indigestion

7 The sounds of peristalsis is normally heard in cattle during auscultation in the lungs areas on the left side, and those sounds are due to movement of

a) Reticulum b) Lungs

c) Abomasum d) Colon

8 Respiratory failure result in

a) Metabolic acidosis b) Metabolic alkalosis
c) Dehydration d) All of the above

9 In geriatric cats, polydipsia and polyuria are common signs of

a) Hyperthyroidism b) Renal failure
c) Diabetes mellitus d) All of the above

10 Pica is the manifestation in deficiency of

a) Phosphorus b) Calcium
c) Molybdenum d) All of the above

11 Vaccine against avian influenza H5N1 strain has been developed by

a) IVRI Mukteshwar b) CSIR
c) HSDAL d) TANUVAS

12 BAER test is used to examine lesions of

a) Optic nerve b) Auditory nerve
c) Recurrent Laryngeal nerve d) None

13 A moderate to severe ketonemia is always present with normal blood sugar level in

a) Diaphragmatic hernia b) Abomasal displacement
c) Vagus indigestion d) Traumatic reticulo peritonitis

14 Most commonly used lead system to record the major electrical force in the heart of the large animal with best amplitude wave form is/are

a) Bipolar lead system b) Unipolar chest leads
c) Both (a) and (b) d) Base-apex monitor lead

15 The specific gravity of isothenuric urine is

a) 1.008-1.012 b) 1.012-1.016
c) 1.001-1.004 d) 1.020-1.030

16 Fluid thrill is perceived in ascites by

a) Auscultation b) Indirect palpation
c) Tactile percussion d) Direct palpation

17 CSF protein is qualitatively detected by

a) Heller's test b) Gemlin test
c) Sulkowitch test d) Pandey's test

18 Metabolic diseases in sheep has greatest significance in

a) Lactating ewes
b) Female sheep during dry period
c) Pregnant ewes
d) Adult sheep

19 Which of the followings is equired for emulsification of dietary fat?

a) Hydrochloric acid
b) Propionic acid
c) Pepsin
d) bile acids

20 What percent solution of Calcium borogluconate is recommended for intravenous infusion in cases of milk fever?

a) 10%
b) 25%
c) 40%
d) 50%

21 Which of the following is liver specific enzyme in cattle

a) SGPT (ALT)
b) SGOT (AST)
c) Sorbitol dehydrogenase
d) Alkaline phosphatase

22 The incidence of milk fever depends on

a) Genetic and management factors
b) Feeding regimen just prior to parturition
c) Breed on the cow
d) All of the above

23 Sampling should be done from following group (s) of animals for the Compton Metabolic profile test

a) Dry cows
b) Medium yielding lactating cows
c) High yielding lactating cows
d) All of the above

24 Ketosis is a metabolic disease that shows signs of

a) Nervous disorder
b) Reduced milk production
c) A typical smell from the mouth
d) All of the above

25 Hemolysis of RBC in nutritional hemoglobinuria is predisposed by deficiency of

a) Zinc
b) Cobalt
c) Selenium
d) Phosphorus

26 Maximum permissible limits of NVLs reactors in a herd for tuberculin testing by single intra-dermal test is

a) 5%
b) 7%
c) 10%
d) 12%

27 A wide spread epidemic that usually affects a large portion of population is called

a) Pandemic b) Endemic

c) Out break d) Trans boundary diseases

28 Who is know as the father of Modern Veterinary Epidemiology?

a) Hippocrates b) Aristotle

c) Thrusfeld d) Alexander Flemmings

29 What is the third component of the epidemiological triad, if the first and second components are host, and agent, respectively?

a) Management b) Breeding practices

c) Environment d) History

30 Usually large numbers of sample sizes are required while investigating a

a) Rare disease. b) Common disease

c) Very common disease d) Pandemic disease

31 The geological structure of an ecosystem may be an important factor in determining the occurrence of following diseases in animals.

a) Mineral deficiency diseases b) Metabolic disesases

c) Vitamin deficiency diseases d) Contagious diseases

32 Any factor responsible for occurrence of the disease is called as

a) Predisposing factor b) Determinant

c) Distant cause d) Secondary cause

33 Endemic form of disease in animal population is termed as

a) Enzootic b) Panzootic

c) Pandemic d) Outbreak

34 Which of the followings reflects the infective power and virulence of the causal factor?

a) Case fatality rate b) Morbidity rate

c) Mortality rate d) Cure rate

35 Actinomycosis may be treated successfully by I/V injection of

a) Potassium Iodide b) Sodium Iodide

c) Tincture Iodine d) Calcium Iodide

36 The common allergic test used for diagnosis of Johne's disease or avian tuberculosis is

a) Single intradermal b) Short thermal test

c) Opthalmic test d) Comparative test

37 The change in milk, generally observed in mastitis is

a) Discoloration b) Presence of clots

c) Presence of flakes d) All of the above

38 Diagnosis of subclinical mastitis depends largely on

a) Clinical signs b) Somatic cell count

c) History d) Age of the animal

39 New castle disease occurs in

a) Chicken b) Ducks

c) Turkeys d) All of the above

40 Rose Bengal test is useful for initial screening of animals for

a) Brucellosis b) Listeriosis

c) Leptospirosis d) Vibriosis

41 Feeding of colostrum provides

a) Passive immunity b) Active immunity

c) Innate immunity d) None of the above

42 Discharge of clear gelatinous exudates from the nodular lesions in the lower limbs is observed in

a) Tuberculosis b) Ulcerative lymphangitis

c) Glanders d) Strangles

43 Rinderpest virus has some antigenic relationship with the virus responsible for

a) Canine distemper b) Foot and Mouth disesae

c) Bovine ephemeral Fever d) Vesicular stomatitis

44 At present, number of FMD virus types are

a) 6 b) 7

c) 8 d) 9

45 FMD does not occur in

a) Cattle b) Horse

c) Goat d) Swine

46 The type of sound produced on palpation of muscles in B.Q is

a) Tympanic b) Crepitating

c) Fluid gurgling sound d) Ping sound

47 In which of the following diseases, post-mortem is generally avoided.

a) Tuberculosis b) Anthrax

c) Brucellosis d) Goat pox

48 The major source of contamination of leptospirosis is

a) Feed material b) Water

c) Urine d) Faecal matter

49 Progressive emaciation, fluctuating temperature and exercise intolerance are salient features of

a) Tuberculosis b) Anthrax

c) Brucellosis d) Goat pox

50 In which form of Ranikhet disease, haemorrhagic lesions are absent and mortality rate is very low

a) Velogenic b) Mesogenic

c) Lentogenic d) None of the above

51 The synonym of Auzjeszky's Disease is

a) Rabies b) Pseudorabies

c) Paratuberculosis d) Infectious Canine hepatitis

52 The more common carrier of leptospirosis is

a) Rodents b) Bats

c) Fishes d) Fomites

53 Fascioliasis may predispose to

a) Black Quarter b) Bacillary haemoglobinuria

c) Anthrax d) Haemorrhagic septicemia

54 Blood may come out with milk during later part of milking in

a) Listeriosis b) Tetanus

c) Botulism d) Tuberculosis

55 Two and half days fever in seen in

a) Strangles b) Paratuberculosis

c) Ephemeral fever d) Infectious bovine Rhinotrachetis

56 Bovine Virus Diarrhoea is caused by

a) Picorna virus b) Adeno virus

c) Pesti virus d) None of the above

57 Hog cholera is caused by

a) Rhabdo virus b) Paramyxo virus

c) Pesti virus d) Toga virus

58 Softness of skull bone, blindness, high stepping gait and paralysis in a sheep are characteristic features of

a) Gid b) Ascariasis

c) Strongyloidosis d) Echinococcosis

59 Pimply gut is caused by

a) *Ascaris suum* b) *Taenia solium*

c) Liver fluke d) *Oesophagostomum columbianum*

60 Rotational grazing of cattle and sheep is recommended to prevent

a) Viral disease b) Parasitic disease

c) Bacterial disease d) Mycoplasma virus

61 *Dirofilaria immitis* generally inhabits in

a) Ventricle b) Bronchi

c) Cerebrum d) Oesophagus

62 *Ascaris suum* commonly affects

a) Dog b) Cat

c) Pig d) Cattle

63 Administration of hyperimmune serum confers

a) Active immunity b) Passive immunity

c) Innate immunity d) Non specific immunity

64 Hyperkeratosis of nose and footpad is a notable feature of

a) Equine distemper b) Canine distemper

c) Equine influenza d) Swine fever

65 Initially, oedema and hyperemia and ultimately atrophy of bursa fabricius is observed in

a) IBR b) ILT

c) IBD d) AIB

66 Botulinum toxin is a

a) Haemolysing toxin b) Neurotoxin

c) Apithliotropic toxin d) All of the above

67 "Tiger-heart" lesion is observed in

a) Strangles b) FMD

c) BEF d) BSE

68 The word not related to the group

a) Calcium b) Vitamin-k

c) Prothrombin d) Analgesics

69 The word not related to the group

a) Lameness b) Bony exostosis

c) Mottling of teeth d) Convulsion

70 The word not related to the group

a) Actinomycosis b) FMD

c) Brucellosis d) Actinobacillosis

71 The word not related to the group

a) Aluminum hydroxide b) Sucralfate

c) Ranitidine d) Berenil

72 The word not related to the group

a) Owners address b) Floor space

c) Past disease d) Line of treatment

73 Accumulation of air in the thoracic cavity is termed as

a) Pneumoperitonium b) Emphysema

c) Pneumothorax d) Pleurisy

74 The nervous disorder manifested by violet activities with little regard to surrounding asseen in rabies is termed as

a) Mania b) Hyperexcitation

c) Frenzy d) Coma

75 Presence of bran like scales on skin surface

a) Wheal b) Pruritus

c) Pityriasis d) Pyoderma

76 Forecasting of a disease is termed as

a) Diagnosis b) Anamnesis

c) Prognosis d) History taking

77 Failure of regeneration of erythrocytes in the bone marrow leads to

a) Aplastic anemia b) Hemolytic anemia

c) Hemorrhagic anemia d) Regenerative anaemia

78 Dehydration in animals can be assessed by

a) PCV b) Skin tenting

c) Total protein d) All of the above

79 Hyperthermia may be seen following feeding of

a) Strychnine b) Eucalypotash

c) Cyanogentic plant d) Legumnous fodder

80 Hyperthermia refers to

a) Elevation of body temperature due totoxemia

b) Elevation of body temperature withouttoxemia

c) Decreased body temperature associated with toxemia

d) Increased body temperature with septicemia

81 Severe acute hemorrhages lead to

a) Congestive heart failure b) Peripheral circulatory failure

c) Anaemic anaemia d) Edema

82 The major site of blood cell formation in post-foetal life

a) Liver b) Spleen

c) Bone marrow d) Thymus

83 Enlargement of prescapular lymph nodes is observed in

a) Babesiosis b) Anthrax

c) Anaplasmosis d) Theileriois

84 In ketosis

a) Acetoacetic acid may increase up to7mg/dl

b) Blood Free fatty acid goes down

c) Beta-hydroxy butyric acid and glucose may remain normal

d) All of the above

85 The deficiency of which of the following vitamins causes star gazing posture and opisthotonus in chicks.

a) Vitamin B1/ Thamine b) Riboflavin

c) Cyanocobalamine d) Niacin

86 Depigmentation of skin in buffaloes and pasty faeces in ruminants is seen in deficiency

a) Cobalt b) Copper

c) Zinc d) Selenium

87 Absorption of magnesium from the GI tract is influenced by

a) Potassium b) Nitrogen

c) Sodium and potassium ratio d) All of the above

88 Deficiency of which of the following hampers the production of RBC

a) Copper b) Iron

c) Cobalt d) All of the above

89 Which of following biomolecules has a direct relationship with protein intake?

a) AST b) Blood creatinine

c) Blood urea nitrogen d) ALT

90 The excess presence of which of the followings in soil causes copper deficiency in cattle?

a) Molybdenum b) Sulfate

c) Both A and B d) Sodium

91 Absorption of magnesium from the GI tract is not influenced by

a) Potassium b) Nitrogen

c) Sodium and potassium ratio d) None of the above

92 Copper deficiency leads to

a) Hypochromic macrocytic anaemia

b) Hypochromic normocytic anaemia

c) Hypochromic microcytic anaemia

d) Hypochromic macrocytic anaemia

93 Secondary copper deficiency occurs due to

a) Reduced level copper in soil

b) Excess of molybdenum in plants/ fodder

c) Reduced intake of protein rich diet

d) Reduced level of sulfate in the soil

94 The possible hypothesis of RBC lysis in post-parturient hemoglobinuria

a) Increased size of the erythrocytes

b) Increased peroxidation of RBCmembrane

c) Decreased malonaldehyde level of erythrocyte membrane
d) Irregular shape of the RBC

95 The typical posture of paralytic myoglobinuria
a) Standing erect
b) Saw-horse posture
c) Attempting to lift the hind quarters
d) Star-gazing position

96 In which case, wound size does not correspond to shape and size of the weapon, the edges of wound are torn and irregular and bleeding may or may not occur and the healing process is very slow
a) Incised wound b) Contused wound
c) Lacerated wound d) Gunshot wound

97 In cases of bestiality, the vaginal washings of the animals is examined for the presence of
a) Human spermatozoa b) Clotted Blood
c) Animal spermatozoa d) Mucus

98 Cruelty to animals include
a) Overloading b) Using diseased animals for work
c) Starvation d) All of the above

99 Which of the followings tantamount to frauds in animal?
a) Castration b) Colouring of the body coat
c) Putting mud in chronic wound d) All of the above

100 Abnormal frequent passage of urine is known as
a) Anuria b) Oliguria
c) Pollakiuria d) Polyurea

Answer Key

1	a	**2**	d	**3**	b	**4**	c	**5**	a	**6**	a	**7**	a	**8**	a	**9**	d	**10**	a
11	c	**12**	b	**13**	b	**14**	c	**15**	a	**16**	c	**17**	d	**18**	c	**19**	d	**20**	b
21	c	**22**	d	**23**	d	**24**	d	**25**	d	**26**	c	**27**	a	**28**	c	**29**	c	**30**	a
31	a	**32**	b	**33**	a	**34**	a	**35**	b	**36**	d	**37**	d	**38**	b	**39**	d	**40**	a
41	a	**42**	b	**43**	a	**44**	b	**45**	b	**46**	b	**47**	b	**48**	c	**49**	a	**50**	c
51	b	**52**	a	**53**	b	**54**	d	**55**	c	**56**	c	**57**	d	**58**	a	**59**	d	**60**	b

61 a	**62** c	**63** b	**64** b	**65** c	**66** b	**67** b	**68** d	**69** d	**70** b
71 d	**72** d	**73** c	**74** c	**75** c	**76** c	**77** a	**78** d	**79** a	**80** b
81 b	**82** c	**83** d	**84** d	**85** a	**86** b	**87** d	**88** d	**89** c	**90** c
91 d	**92** c	**93** b	**94** b	**95** b	**96** c	**97** a	**98** d	**99** d	**100** b

31

Miscellaneous Exercise VI

1 Ovine ketosis is more common during

a) Early lactation b) Late Pregnancy

c) Early Pregnancy d) Late lactation

2 An example for positive ionotropic drug is

a) Isoproterenol b) Amlodipin

c) Enalapril d) Chlorthalidone

3 Baby pig disease is characterized by

a) Hypocalcaemia b) Hypoglycemia

c) Hypothyroidism d) Hypopituitarism

4 Which one of the following is required for the conversion of T4 to T3

a) Zinc b) Manganese

c) Copper d) Selenium

5 Severe proteinuria occurs in

a) Glomerular disease b) Renal amyloidosis

c) UTI d) Urolithiasis

6 The preferred parenteral fluid for treatment of bovine ruminal acidosis is

a) DNS b) 5D

c) RL d) Haemaccel

7 In toxaemia, there is

a) Fall in blood sugar level b) Increase in blood sugar level

c) Blood sugar not altered d) Hypothermia

8 Parakeratosis of skin in pigs is noticed due to deficiency of

a) Zinc b) Copper

c) Cobalt d) Iron

9 The specific drug used for gastric ulcer is

a) Belladona b) Sucralfate

c) Kaolin d) Ranitidine

10 Abdominal fluid thrill in ascites in dogs can be detected by

a) Auscultation b) Indirect palpation

c) Tactile percussion d) Direct palpation

11 Haemoglobinuria associated with hepatitis is common in

a) Cattle b) Sheep

c) Horses d) Pigs

12 Man satisfying his lust through an animal is termed as

a) Sodomy b) Lesbianism

c) Bestiality d) Tribadism

13 Upper motor neuron disease causes

a) Flaccid paralysis b) Spastic Paralysis

c) Hemiparesis d) Paresis

14 Pin point to echymotic subconjunctival haemorrhages in bovines is seen in

a) Toxemia b) Septicemia

c) Conjunctivitis d) Hypothermia

15 In hyperthermia, increased thirst is due to

a) High environmental temperature

b) Profused sweating

c) Loss of sodium chloride from the body

d) Dryness of the mouth

16 The normal ruminal pH of bovines fed with both concentrates and roughages is

a) 6.5-7.0 b) 5.5-6.5

c) 6.8-7.2 d) 7.2-8.2

17 Photosensitization is a feature of poisoning with

a) Datura b) Lantana

c) Abrus d) Bracken fern

18 The most effective drug for the treatment of anaphylactic shock is

a) Atropine sulphate b) Digoxine

c) Epinephrine d) Dopamine

19 Eclampsia in bitches is best treated with

a) 50% Dextrose b) 10% Calcium gluconate

c) Thiamine d) Mifex

20 Highest incidence of Lactation tetany in mares is seen

a) 1-2 days after weaning b) 10 days after weaning

c) 20 days after weaning d) 30 days after weaning

21 Downer cow like syndrome can be a complication of

a) Dystocia b) Mastitis

c) Metrititis d) Tympany

22 Transition period in dairy cows is

a) 8 weeks before to 8 weeks after parturition

b) 5 weeks before to 5 weeks after parturition

c) 3 weeks before to 3 weeks after parturition

d) 1 week before to 1 week after parturition

23 Ischemic myopathy is a feature of

a) Sodium deficiency b) Weak Calf syndrome

c) Downer cow syndrome d) Milk fever

24 Laryngitis in dogs can be observed in

a) Canine Distemper b) ICH

c) Parvovirus d) Rabies

25 The B Complex vitamin having potential gluconeogenic and antilypolytic activity is

a) Riboflavin b) Thiamine

c) Niacin d) Pyridoxine

26 The biochemical alteration that occurs in toxaemia is

a) Low blood glucose level b) Low blood NPN

c) Low total serum protein d) High creatinine level

27 Ideal antidote for arrhythmia associated with intravenous calcium toxicity

a) Adrenaline b) Atropine

c) Pilocarpin d) Neostigmine

28 The traumatic reticulo pericarditis is characterized by

a) Shift to left b) Shift to right

c) Leukopenia d) Neutropenia

29 The short chain fatty acid synthesized in the rumen with highest glucogenic activity

a) Acetic acid
b) Propionic acid
c) Butyric acid
d) Lactic acid

30 Excess dietary supplementation of which of the following minerals interferes in the absorption of Fluorine?

a) Sodium
b) Potassium
c) Calcium
d) Iodine

31 The preferred fluid for treatment of ruminal acidosis is

a) DNS
b) RL
c) Haemaccel
d) NSS

32 Rapid fall in body temperature of an animal is termed as

a) Crisis
b) Lysis
c) Hypothermia
d) Hyperthermia

33 Biological precursor for Co-enzyme A used for the treatment of bovine ketosis is

a) Vebonal
b) Cysteamine
c) Monensin
d) Trembolone

34 Which of the following infectious diseases of dog has got a zoonotic importance?

a) Canine hepatitis
b) Canine Distemper
c) Canine leptospirosis
d) Corona virus infection

35 The most useful anionic compound for prevention of milk fever in cattle is

a) Sodium Chloride
b) Potassium Chloride
c) Ammonium chloride
d) Calcium chloride

36 Ping sound on simultaneous percussion and auscultation is characteristic of

a) Simple indigestion
b) Acid indigestion
c) Left side abomasal displacement
d) Vagus indigestion

37 Type of fever in canine distemper is

a) Biphagic fever
b) Atypical fever
c) Intermittent fever
d) Recurrent fever

38 Commonly used cytoprotectant in the treatment of gastric ulcer is

a) Ondansetron b) Metoclopramide

c) Sucralfate d) Tannic acid

39 High plasma cortisol level is a feature of

a) Bovine ketosis b) Ovine ketosis

c) Milk fever d) Eclampsia

40 Vitamin that protects the cellular membranes from lipid peroxidation is

a) Vitamin-A b) Vitamin-D

c) Vitamin-E d) Vitamin-K

41 Lactation tetany in mare is caused by

a) Hypoglycemia b) Hypocalcemia

c) Hypophosphataemia d) Hypomagnesemia

42 Significant elevation of which enzyme is diagnostic of Downer cow syndrome

a) Alkaline phosphatase b) Alanine aminotransferase

c) Creatinine phosphokinase d) Gamma glutamyl transpeptidase

43 Uraemia in dog is often accompanied by

a) Vomiting b) Fever

c) Abdominal Pain d) Ascites

44 Cattle that are not exposed to ultraviolet solar radiation are prone to the deficiency of

a) Vitamin-A b) Vitamin-D

c) Vitamin-E d) Vitamin-K

45 The area for auscultation of heart is

a) 3-5 intercoastal space b) 2-3 intercoastal space

c) 5-6 intercoastal space d) 12-13 intercoastal space

46 Canine atopic dermatitis can be diagnosed by blood sample examination for the level of

a) Eisonophil b) IgE

c) IgM d) Neutrophil

47 Heavy application of nitrogen fertilizer in soil enhances the soil concentration of

a) Copper b) Cobalt

c) Magnesium d) Molybdenum

48 Secondary iodine deficiency is usually caused by

a) High Cu intake
b) Hypervitaminosis A
c) High Ca intake
d) Reduced sodium intake

49 Abnormal utilization of Vit-E has a sparing effect on

a) Vit-A
b) Essential fatty Acids
c) Thiamine
d) Molybdenum

50 Minimum daily requirement of vit-A /kg bwt in bovines is

a) 440 IU
b) 200 IU
c) 40 IU
d) 3000 IU

51 Which clinical symptom may not develop due to potassium deficiency in calves?

a) Poor growth
b) Anaemia
c) Diarrhoea
d) Muscular weakness

52 Pleural and peritoneal effusions in cats are seen in

a) Feline panleukemia
b) Feline Infectious peritonitis
c) Rabies
d) Oesophagitis

53 Which mineral deficiency may cause acute heart failure

a) Copper
b) Selenium
c) Both Copper & Selenium
d) Zinc

54 Drug of choice for treatment of Endocarditis

a) Penicillin
b) Chloramphenicol
c) Gentamycin
d) Tetracyclin

55 Atrophic gastritis in piglets is caused due to the deficiency of

a) Copper
b) Manganese
c) Calcium
d) Iron

56 P wave in ECG indicates

a) Atrial depolarization
b) Ventricular depolarization
c) ventricular repolarisation
d) Atrial repolarization

57 Non inflammatory degeneration of skeletal muscle is known as

a) Myasthenia
b) Myopathy
c) Myositis
d) Muscular atrophy

58 The most toxic grain for causing ruminal acidosis is

a) Oat b) Sorghum

c) Barley d) Bajra

59 Shock that occurs when there is reduction in circulating blood volume is called

a) Haemorrhagic shock b) Hypovolemic shock

c) Septic shock d) Obstructive shock

60 Osteodystrophia fibrosa or bran disease occurs in horses fed on high level of

a) Phosphorus b) Calcium

c) Vit. D d) Magnesium

61 Drug of choice against Bovine Fascioliasis is

a) Triquin b) Triclabendazole

c) Levamisole d) Pyrantel embonate

62 Valvular disease is mainly characterised by presence of

a) Friction sound b) Murmurs

c) Gallop sound d) Box sound

63 White muscle disease is caused by

a) Excess of selenium

b) Excess of vit-C

c) Deficiency of vitamin-E or selenium

d) Abnormal synthesis of vitamin-D

64 Digitalis is contraindicated in

a) Dilated cardiomyopathy b) Ventricular tachycardia

c) Restrictive cardiomyopathy d) Congestive heart failure

65 Ovine white liver disease has been recorded in sheep due to the deficiency of

a) Copper b) Cobalt

c) Zinc d) Iron

66 Making the animals useless by means of violence

a) Bishoping b) Maiming

c) Cruelty d) Bestiality

67 Wool-eating symptom is commonly noticed in sheep due to deficiency of

a) Calcium b) Phosphorous

c) Vit-D d) Zinc

68 Hypersecretory diarrhoea in neonatal farm animals is caused by

a) *Streptococcous* b) *Pseudomonas*

c) *E. coli* d) *Klebsiella* sp.

69 Hypoprotenemia and subcutaneous oedema are commonly noticed in

a) Abomasitis b) Parasitic Enteritis

c) Both of the above d) Urea feeding

70 Drug of choice for status epilepticus

a) Diazepam I/M b) Diazepam orally

c) Phenobarbitone d) Primidone

71 Intense icterus is noticed in case of

a) Parvo virus infection b) Leptospirosis

c) Canine distemper d) Ehrlichosis

72 Specific test used for diagnosis of cardiomyopathy

a) Troponin I b) SGPT

c) SGOT d) GGT

73 Canine parvo virus can be diagnosed from fecal sample through

a) Microscopic examination b) PCR

c) FAT d) All of the above

74 Fluid of choice for cerebral oedema

a) Dextrose 5% b) 20% Mannitol solution

c) RL d) DNS

75 Total number of essential amino acids in dogs are

a) 10 b) 11

c) 12 d) 13

76 An example for endocrinopathy of dog with multiple neurologic manifestations

a) Hypoadrenocorticism b) Hypothyroidism

c) Hyperthyroidism d) Hyperoestrogenism

77 The best information required for breeding of dogs is

a) Pedigree b) Individual

c) Family d) Sibs

78 Horizontal nystagmus is the characteristic sign of

a) Peripheral vestibular disease b) Central vestibular disease

c) Mental abnormalities d) Spondilitis

79 Infectious disease of dog having no zoonotic importance is

a) Infectious Canine hepatitis b) Rabies

c) Canine leptospirosis d) Listeriosis

80 The dog breed very prone to inherited cerebellar hypoplasia is

a) Irish setter b) GSD

c) Dalmatian d) Pug

81 A vaccination certificate issued by a veterinarian is required for

a) Sale of animal

b) Maintenance of pet

c) Transportation across the state border

d) Protection of pet against diseases

82 Most common cause of lameness in adult dairy cow is

a) selenium toxicosis b) Warts

c) Laminitis d) Sub solar disease

83 The legal aspects related to veterinary profession and different livestock are covered in

a) Veterinary jurisprudence b) Veterinary medicine

c) Veterinary toxicology d) Veterinary Clinical Medicine

84 Occulo cardiac reflex is used to assess the function of

a) Vagus nerve b) Optic nerve

c) Trigeminal nerve d) Vestibular nerve

85 The sample stored for vetero-legal examination can be kept for a period of maximum

a) 1 year b) 2 months

c) 6 months d) 15 days

86 Softening of mature bone

a) Rickets b) Osteomalacia

c) Osteoperosis d) Osteodystrophic fibrosa

87 Simple method for assessing bone marrow activity in anaemic patient

a) RBC count b) WBC count

c) DLC d) Reticulocyte count

88 Contused wounds are produced by

a) Bullet b) Sword

c) Nail d) Whip

89 Name one enzyme deficiency which cause haemolytic anaemia in dog

a) Pyruvate kinase b) CPK

c) Erythropoietin d) Transketolase

90 Which diet may accelerate the formation of calcium phosphate calculi in the bladder and kidney

a) Low vitamin - A and high Calcium

b) Low vitamin - A and low calcium

c) High vitamin - A and high calcium

d) High vitamin - A and low calcium

91 Kangaroo sitting position in pigs is due to the deficiency of

a) Riboflavin b) Pantothenic acid

c) Niacin d) Biotin

92 Star grazing posture in chickens are found in deficiency of

a) Vitamin-A b) Thiamine

c) Vitamin-E & Se d) Cyanocobalamin

93 Short ferky inspiration caused by stimulation of Phrenic nerve is called

a) Hiccough b) Wheeze

c) Roar d) Sneezing

94 A high incidence of stillbirth is recorded in the litters of sows suffering from

a) Copper deficiency b) Zinc deficiency

c) Cobalt deficiency d) Iron deficiency anaemia

95 In dogs, excessive barking leads to

a) Bronchitis b) Laryngitis

c) Trachietis d) Pharyngitis

96 The young succulent rapid growing pasture has high concentration of

a) Potassium b) Magnesium

c) Carbohydrate d) Phosphorous

97 Peat scours occurs in calves due to

a) Presence of sulphate in the diet b) Lack of molybdate in the diet

c) Deficiency of zinc in the diet d) Excess molybdenum in the diet

98 Death in post parturient hemoglobinurea occurs due to

a) Decubital septicaemia b) Anemic anoxia

c) Myocarditis d) uremia

99 Thin soft skin in a characteristic feature in

a) Hypothyroidism b) Hyperadrenocorticism

c) Hyperoestrogenism d) Pemphigus vulgaris

100 The hemolytic factor present in cabbage is

a) Thiouracil b) Thiocyanate

c) Thiosulphate d) Gossypol

Answer Key

1	b	**2**	c	**3**	b	**4**	d	**5**	b	**6**	c	**7**	a	**8**	a	**9**	b	**10**	c
11	c	**12**	c	**13**	b	**14**	b	**15**	d	**16**	b	**17**	b	**18**	c	**19**	b	**20**	a
21	a	**22**	c	**23**	c	**24**	c	**25**	c	**26**	a	**27**	b	**28**	a	**29**	b	**30**	c
31	b	**32**	a	**33**	b	**34**	c	**35**	c	**36**	c	**37**	a	**38**	c	**39**	b	**40**	c
41	d	**42**	c	**43**	a	**44**	b	**45**	a	**46**	d	**47**	d	**48**	c	**49**	a	**50**	c
51	b	**52**	b	**53**	c	**54**	a	**55**	d	**56**	a	**57**	b	**58**	a	**59**	b	**60**	a
61	b	**62**	b	**63**	c	**64**	b	**65**	b	**66**	b	**67**	d	**68**	a	**69**	c	**70**	c
71	b	**72**	a	**73**	d	**74**	b	**75**	a	**76**	b	**77**	a	**78**	a	**79**	a	**80**	a
81	c	**82**	c	**83**	a	**84**	a	**85**	c	**86**	b	**87**	b	**88**	d	**89**	a	**90**	a
91	d	**92**	b	**93**	a	**94**	d	**95**	b	**96**	a	**97**	d	**98**	b	**99**	b	**100**	a

32

Miscellaneous Exercise VII

1 Hepatosis dietetica in swine is caused by

a) Deficiency of vitamin-E & Se

b) Feeding of high energy diet

c) Excess of unsaturated fatty acid in the diet

d) Deficiency of vitamin A

2 Ketosis should be differentiated from

a) Louping ill b) Listeriosis

c) Otitis d) Milk fever

3 Oral thrush in birds is caused by

a) *Pasteurella multocida* b) *Salmonella enterliticum*

c) *Candidia albicans* d) Fowl pox

4 Drug of choice for treating Ehrlichiosis in canine is

a) Imidocarb b) Quinapyramine

c) Morentel d) Piperazine

5 Important zoonotic disease from cat is

a) Scabies b) Toxoplasmosis,

c) Listeriosis d) Leptospirosis

6 Type of diabetes mellitus commonly occurs in dogs is

a) Insulin independent b) Insulin dependent

c) Pregnancy diabetes d) Congenital diabetes

7 Monocytosis in dogs is a characteristic feature in

a) Ehrlichilosis b) Anaplasmosis

c) Babesiosis d) Parvovirus infection

8 Chorea with repeated epileptic episode in dogs is characteristic sign in

a) Canine distemper b) Canine Parvo

c) Lyme's Disease d) Canine hepatitis

9 Parakeratosis in swine is due to

a) Zn deficiency b) Unsaturated fatty acid deficiency
c) Inherited factors d) Copper deficiency

10 The objectives of fluid therapy in diarrhoea is to correct

a) Dehydration b) Alkalosis
c) Glucose deficiency d) Protein deficiency

11 The objectives of fluid therapy in Haemorrhage is to prevent

a) Dehydration b) Alkalosis
c) Hypovolumic shock d) Acidosis

12 In traumatic reticulo pericarditis there will be

a) Neutrophillia b) Eosinophillia
c) Lymphocytosis d) Leukocytopenia

13 Regular consumption of raw fish by dogs results in deficiency of

a) Riboflavin b) Thiamine
c) Zinc d) Manganese

14 Typical bruits on auscultation indicates

a) Endocarditis b) Pericarditis
c) Pericardial effusion d) None

15 Yellow fat disease in kitten is due to deficiency of

a) Vitamin-E b) Vitamin-A
c) Vitamin-C d) Iodine

16 The common alterations in blood noticed in toxaemia of bacterial origin

a) Increased total serum protein b) Increased blood NPN
c) Low blood glucose d) Neutrophillia

17 Type of anoxia in HCN poisoning is

a) Stagnant anoxia b) Histotoxic anoxia
c) Anaemic anoxia d) Anoxic anoxia

18 Simple indigestion is to be differentiated from

a) Vagus indigestion b) RDA
c) Heat stroke d) Caecal impaction

19 Steatorrhoea is a feature for dysfunction of

a) Kidney b) Liver

c) Heart d) Spleen

20 The distension of the lungs caused by over distension of the alveoli with rupture of alveolar walls and escape of air into the interstitial spaces is termed as

a) Pulmonary oedema b) Pulmonary congestion

c) Pulmonary emphysema d) Hydrothorax

21 Secondary iodine deficiency is usually caused by

a) High Cu intake b) Hypervitaminosis A

c) High Ca intake d) High Na intake

22 The first organ to be affected during hypoxic condition in animals

a) Kidney b) Heart

c) Liver d) Brain

23 Minimum daily requirement of Vit. A/kg.bwt in all species is

a) 440 IU b) 200 IU

c) 40 IU d) 3000IU

24 The most common feature noticed in toxaemia is

a) Hypoglycemia b) Glycosuria

c) Low serum protein d) Low blood NPN

25 Parakeratosis in swine is due to

a) Zn deficiency b) Unsaturated fatty acid deficiency

c) Inherited factors d) Sodium deficiency

26 In viral pneumonia, the blood CBC picture shows

a) Neutropenia b) Lymphocytosis

c) Both of the above d) Monocytosis

27 Calcium deficiency in animals can be detected by

a) Estimation of Methylmalonic acid

b) Estimation of Formiminoglutamic acid

c) Vit. B12 level in the body

d) Salkowitch test

28 Nutritional hepatitis is also known as

a) Toxic hepatitis
b) Trophopathic hepatitis
c) Infectious hepatitis
d) Obstructive hepatitis

29 Which type of wound generally has two openings

a) incised wound
b) Contused wound
c) Lacerated wound
d) Gunshot wound

30 Acute hepatic failure in goats is manifested by

a) Diarrhoea
b) Submandibular oedema
c) Steatorrhoea
d) Constipation

31 Goitre in kids is due to deficiency of

a) Vit.E
b) Vit.A
c) Vit.C
d) Iodine

32 In cyclo-oxygenase pathway, which of the following metabolites is produced from arachidonic acid?

a) Thromboxane A2
b) Leukotrine
c) Prostraglandin
d) Parathormone

33 The normal serum total protein concentration in dogs is

a) 6-8 gm/dl
b) 4 - 5 gm/dl
c) 8-12gm/dl
d) 13-15gm/dl

34 Adulteration of sesame oil in ghee is detected by

a) Phytostryl Acetate test
b) Boudouin test
c) Stoch test
d) Iodine test

35 The normal albumin and globulin ration in dogs is

a) 0.4
b) 0.5
c) 0.9
d) 1.2

36 Malpractice in livestock sale is punishable under section

a) IPC 420
b) IPC 440
c) IPC 320
d) IPC 220

37 In obstructive jaundice, the colour of the faeces is

a) Brownish green
b) Tarry black
c) Dark coloured
d) Clay coloured

38 The approximate energy content on dry matter basis in dog food should be

a) 3300-4000 kcal/kg b) 5500-6000 kcal

c) 2300-3000 kcal/kg d) 4300-5000 kcal/kg

39 Partial loss of appetite is known as

a) Inappetence b) Anorexia

c) Anaphagia d) Dysphagia

40 Which of the following is a long haired dog breed

a) Basset hound b) Afghan hound

c) Grey hound d) Rampur hound

41 Anamnesis refers to as recording of

a) Clinical signs b) History taking

c) General inspection d) Palpation

42 The aminoacids which is highly essential to be incorpotated in cat feed is

a) Lysine b) Taurine

c) Isoleusin d) Arginine

43 Abducted elbows and careful gait are associated with

a) Vagus indigestion b) Traumatic reticulo pericarditis

c) RDA d) Ruminal acidosis

44 In medico-legal cases, the veterinarian is requested by the police authorities for assisting them in

a) Diagnosis b) Legal proceedings

c) Transportation of the animals d) Treatment

45 Enlargement of mediastinal lymph node in cattle results in

a) Frothy bloat b) Constipation

c) Free gas bloat d) None of the above

46 Reduced oxygen carrying capacity of the blood occurring in carbon monoxide poisoning is a type of

a) Anoxic anoxia b) Histotoxic anoxia

c) Anaemic anoxia d) Stagnent anoxia

47 Epistaxis can be treated with

a) Vit-E b) Vit - B1

c) Vit-C d) Vit-K

48 Ascites in dogs may occur due to failure of

a) Lungs b) Brain

c) Kidney d) Spleen

49 The most common type of fever in Veterinary practice

a) Intermittent b) Atypical

c) Relapsing d) Undulant

50 The constitution of India provides animal protection by

a) Article 51 b) Article 52

c) Article 53 d) Article 54

51 The primary modes or causes of death include

a) Ascites b) Fever

c) Asphyxia d) Hepatic encephalopathy

52 The wild life protection act was drafted and implemented in year

a) 1962 b) 1972

c) 1982 d) 1992

53 Mischief is punishable under the section

a) IPC 377 b) . IPC-420

c) Both (a) and (b) d) IPC 379

54 The trypanosomiasis in camel is known as

a) Tribursa b) Surra

c) Bibarsa d) Circling diseases

55 Lack of fluid intake leads to

a) Oedema

b) Catabolism of fat, protein andcarbohydrate

c) No effect on tissue fluid level

d) Increase in fluid output

56 The clinical signs of dyspnoea is

a) Open mouth breathing b) Retraction of tongue

c) Decreased depth of respiration d) All of the above

57 In hepatic jaundice, there is increase in serum level of

a) Unconjugated billirubin b) Conjugated billirubin

c) Both (a) and (b) d) Billiverdin

58 In viral pneumonia in cat, the blood picture shows

a) Neutrophilia b) Leucocytosis

c) Lymphocytopenia d) Monocytosis

59 The minimum serum billirubin concentration for clinically evident icterus in animal is

a) 1 mg/dl b) 2 mg/dl

c) 0.5 mg/dl d) 5 mg/dl

60 Hypocalcemia in a high yielding cow cause

a) Primary bloat b) Secondary bloat

c) Both a and b d) Forthy boat

61 The emulsifier used in the treatment of ruminal tympany is

a) Pleuronic L64 b) Magnesium sulphate

c) Dioctyol sodium sulfosuccinate d) Monensin

62 Bestiality comes under section

a) 272 b) 193

c) 377 d) 437

63 In ruminal bloat, the stability of foam increases at the pH

a) above 7.5 b) Between 7 to 6

c) 6 or below d) 8.5

64 Doping test is done

a) Race horse b) Cat

c) Dog d) Camel

65 In abomasal impaction of cattle, there is

a) Hypokalemia b) Hyperchloremia

c) Hypophosphatemia d) Hyponatremia

66 The increased amylase and lipase level in peritoneal fluid of dogs than that of serum indicates

a) Obstructive jaundice b) Hepatitis

c) Pancreatitis d) Nephritis

67 In E.C.G, P wave represents

a) Arterial depolarisation b) Ventricular repolarisation

c) Atrial repolarisation d) Ventricular depolarisation

68 Hydrothorax in animals may occur in

a) Pancreatic disorder b) Vagus nerve injury

c) Hypoproteinemia d) RFA

69 The condition in which the bacteria remains in circulation throughout the disease process and produces clinical signs is

a) Bacteremia b) Septicemia

c) Viremia d) Toxemia

70 The type of sub mucosal and sub conjunctival haemorrhages seen in conjunctiva of eye, mouth and vulva in septicemia is

a) Extensive b) Petechial

c) Both (a) and (b) d) Localized

71 The choice of drug for treatment of ruminal alkalosis is

a) Acetic acid b) Ascorbic acid

c) Hydrochloric acid d) Sodium Bicarbonate

72 In simple indigestion, ruminal pH remains in the range of

a) 4.5-5.0 b) 5.1-5.9

c) 6.0-7.0 d) 8.0-9.0

73 In ruminal acidosis, the alkalinizer used to correct ruminal pH is

a) Magnesium hydroxide b) Sodium bicarbonate

c) Epsom salt d) Calcium chloride

74 Post parturient haemoglobinuria is predisposed by deficiency of

a) Cobalt b) Magnesium

c) Phosphorus d) Zinc

75 First stage of milk fever in cattle is identified by

a) Excitement and tetany b) Sitting on the sternum

c) No pupilary light reflex d) None of the above

76 Alimentary ketosis in cattle occur due to the silage containing

a) Excessive butyrates b) Low butyrates

c) High oxalets d) Low propionates

77 Post parturient hemoglobinuria occurs due to

a) Copper deficiency b) Phosphorous deficiency

c) Potassium deficiency d) Cobalt deficiency

78 Cardioscopy is a

a) Invasive method b) Non Invasive method

c) Intense-invasive method d) Semi-invasive method

79 The toxic product present in plants belonging to crucifera family and responsible for causing haemolysis is

a) Thiouracil b) Thyocil

c) Uremic acid d) Gossypol

80 Milk fever is detected biochemically through

a) Benedicts test b) Sulphur granule test

c) Sulkowitch test d) Rothera test

81 Vigorous licking of skin & inanimate object is seen in

a) Nervous form of ketosis b) Hypomagnesemic tetany

c) Eclampsia d) Pregnancy toxaemia

82 Coagulation of muscle protein & coagulation necrosis of muscle fibre is seen in

a) Grass tetany b) Eclampsia

c) Monday morning sickness d) Downer cow syndrome

83 "Creepers cow" are seen in animals affected with

a) Milk fever b) Ketosis

c) Grass tetany d) Downer cow syndrome

84 Clinical signs of fatty cow syndrome are

a) Ketonuria b) Scanty and firm faeces

c) Both (a) and (b) d) No effect on milk yield

85 The Gold Standard test for the diagnosis of Leptospirosis is

a) Microscopic Agglutination b) AGPT

c) ELISA d) Intradermal hypersensitivity test

86 Parvovirus replicate rapidly in the cells of

a) Intestine b) Lungs

c) Liver d) Skin

87 Coffee coloured urine in a cow is characteristic sign of

a) Babesiosis b) Parvoviral enteritis

c) Ehrlichiosis d) Scabies

88 Lagomorpha comprises of

a) Parraots b) Cats

c) Rabbits d) Reptiles

89 Feeding high calcium diet during pregnancy in dogs can predispose to

a) Pyoderma b) Pneumonia

c) Eclampsia d) Mammitis

90 Pseudopregnancy is more common in

a) Cats b) Rabbits

c) Bitches d) Sows

91 Auscultation of heart during right side congestive heart failure gives

a) Cardiac murmur b) Systolic murmur

c) Both of (a) and (b) d) Friction rub

92 Pulmonary vein congestion seen in which side of cardiac failure

a) Right side b) Left side

c) Either side d) No effect on pulmonary vein

93 Which of the following adult parasite localizes in the nodules in esophageal wall in dog?

a) *Spirocerca lupi* b) *Dictyophylla renale*

c) *Toxocara canis* d) *Ascaris sum*

94 Type of hypoxia causing insufficient oxygenation of arterial blood

a) Hypoxic hypoxia b) Anaemic hypoxia

c) Ischemic hypoxia d) histotoxic hypoxia

95 Doxycycline drugs intoxication in calves causes

a) Pulmonary congestion b) Pulmonary pleurisy

c) Pulmonary emphysema d) Pulmonary oedema

96 Death in cows suffering from postparturient haemoglobinuria is due to

a) Anaemic anoxia b) Histotoxic anoxia

c) Heart failure d) Brain failure

97 Sweetish foetid breath smell may be observed in which type of pneumonia

a) Aspiration pneumonia b) Mycotic pneumonia

c) viral pneumonia d) Parasitic pneumonia

98 Increase in eosinophil count occurs in which type of pneumonia

a) Bacterial b) Parasite

c) Aspiration d) Mycotic

99 Prevention of cruelty to animals act came into existence in year

a) 1960 b) 1980

c) 1970 d) 1950

100 Macrocytic anaemia is seen in deficiency of

a) Iron b) Copper

c) Cobalt d) Selenium

Answer Key

1	a	**2**	b	**3**	c	**4**	a	**5**	b	**6**	b	**7**	a	**8**	a	**9**	a	**10**	a
11	c	**12**	a	**13**	d	**14**	c	**15**	b	**16**	d	**17**	b	**18**	a	**19**	b	**20**	c
21	c	**22**	d	**23**	c	**24**	a	**25**	a	**26**	b	**27**	d	**28**	b	**29**	d	**30**	b
31	d	**32**	c	**33**	b	**34**	a	**35**	b	**36**	a	**37**	d	**38**	a	**39**	a	**40**	b
41	b	**42**	b	**43**	b	**44**	a	**45**	c	**46**	c	**47**	d	**48**	c	**49**	b	**50**	a
51	d	**52**	b	**53**	b	**54**	a	**55**	b	**56**	d	**57**	c	**58**	c	**59**	b	**60**	b
61	a	**62**	c	**63**	a	**64**	a	**65**	b	**66**	c	**67**	a	**68**	c	**69**	b	**70**	b
71	a	**72**	c	**73**	b	**74**	c	**75**	a	**76**	a	**77**	b	**78**	b	**79**	a	**80**	c
81	a	**82**	c	**83**	d	**84**	c	**85**	a	**86**	a	**87**	a	**88**	c	**89**	c	**90**	c
91	b	**92**	b	**93**	a	**94**	a	**95**	d	**96**	a	**97**	a	**98**	b	**99**	a	**100**	c